Judith Ochshorn, PhD
Ellen Cole, PhD
Editors

Women's Spirituality, Women's Lives

Pre-publication
REVIEWS,
COMMENTARIES,
EVALUATIONS . . .

Women's Spirituality, Women's Lives is a delightful and complex book on spirituality and sacredness in women's lives. This book touches on many of the varying approaches that woman has taken in her relationship with Spirit. Readers will be familiarized with myriad ideologies–spanning the globe, the ages, and the female consciousness. This selective collection provides great insight into the vast diversity of woman's approaches to divinity.

Joan Clingan, M.A.
Spiritual Psychology and Education,
Graduate Advisor, Prescott College
Master of Arts Program, Graduate
Assistant, University of Santa Monica

Nothing is more compelling than hearing women speak in their own strong voices. Creating a women's spirituality is a powerful collective experience and a deeply personal process. What makes this anthology so compelling is that it is so intensely personal. Before going on to reflect, critique and analyze their religious experience, Jewish Womanist, Wiccan, Catholic, lesbian, Puerto Rican and Native Americans speak confessionally about their religious practices. The result is that the reader experiences simultaneously the amazing diversity of women's spiritualities and the power of the commonalities created when traditions become women-centered. A wonderful fusion of spiritual practice, psychotherapeutic insight and feminist theologizing melded together through women's distinctive ways of experiencing the divine.

Karen J. Torjesen
Margo H. Goldsmith Chair of Women's Studies in Religion, Claremont Graduate School

In *Women's Spirituality, Women's Lives,* Judith Ochshorn and Ellen Cole have brought together a wide-ranging collection of materials on the healing and empowering aspects of women's religious experience. In stories, poems, essays, interviews, and letters, the authors explore contemporary women's spirituality from a number of perspectives: a Puerto-Rican mother and daughter, a feminist martial arts academy, an African-American Holiness church leader and social activist, a Jewish feminist community, a group of German women seeking to rediscover the roots of spirituality in their own traditions, and many others. These essays often discuss the experimentation of women's groups with new ritual, but also include an empassioned plea for maintaining the integrity of Native American women's religious traditions against the pressures of US consumerist and colonizing attitudes. Out of this rich diversity comes a collective wisdom that affirms the healing power of women's spirituality based on the agency and actions of women coming together for ritual, reflection, and renewal.

Karen L. King, PhD
Associate Professor of Religious Studies, Occidental College

Women's Spirituality, Women's Lives

Women's Spirituality, Women's Lives

Judith Ochshorn, PhD
Ellen Cole, PhD
Editors

The Haworth Press, Inc.
New York • London

The development, preparation, and publication of this work has been undertaken with great care. However, the publisher, employees, editors, and agents of The Haworth Press and all imprints of The Haworth Press, Inc., including the Haworth Medical Press and Pharmaceutical Products Press, are not responsible for any errors contained herein or for consequenses that may ensue from use of materials or information contained in this work. Opinions expressed by the author(s) are not necessarily those of The Haworth Press, Inc.

The Haworth Press, Inc., 10 Alice Street, Binghamton, NY 13904-1580, USA

Library of Congress Cataloging-in-Publication Data

Women's spirituality, women's lives / Judith Ochshorn, Ellen Cole, editors.
    p. cm.
    "Has also been published as Women & therapy, volume 16, numbers 2/3, 1995"–T.p. verso.
    Includes bibliographical references.
    ISBN 1-56024-722-3 -- ISBN 1-56023-065-7
    1. Women--Religious life. 2. Women and religion. I. Ochshorn, Judith, 1928- . II. Cole, Ellen.
BL625.7.W655 1995
248.8'43–dc20   95-11386
                                                          CIP

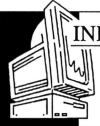

INDEXING & ABSTRACTING

Contributions to this publication are selectively indexed or abstracted in print, electronic, online, or CD-ROM version(s) of the reference tools and information services listed below. This list is current as of the copyright date of this publication. See the end of this section for additional notes.

- *Abstracts of Research in Pastoral Care & Counseling*, Loyola College, 7135 Minstrel Way, Suite 101, Columbia, MD 21045

- *Academic Abstracts/CD-ROM,* EBSCO Publishing, P.O. Box 2250, Peabody, MA 01960-7250

- *Academic Index (on-line)*, Information Access Company, 362 Lakeside Drive, Foster City, CA 94404

- *Alternative Press Index*, Alternative Press Center, Inc., P.O. Box 33109, Baltimore, MD 21218-0401

- *Current Contents: Social & Behavioral Sciences (CC/S & BS)* (weekly Table of Contents Service), and *Social Science Citation Index*. Articles also searchable through *Social SciSearch,* ISI's online database and in ISI's *Research Alert* current awareness service, Institute for Scientific Information, 3501 Market Street, Philadelphia, PA 19104-3302

- *Digest of Neurology and Psychiatry,* The Institute of Living, 400 Washington Street, Hartford, CT 06106

- *Expanded Academic Index,* Information Access Company, 362 Lakeside Drive, Forest City, CA 94404

- *Family Violence & Sexual Assault Bulletin*, Family Violence & Sexual Assault Institute, 1310 Clinic Drive, Tyler, TX 75701

- *Feminist Periodicals: A Current Listing of Contents*, Women's Studies Librarian-at-Large, 728 State Street, 430 Memorial Library, Madison, WI 53706

- *Higher Education Abstracts*, Claremont Graduate School, 740 North College Avenue, Claremont, CA 91711

- *Index to Periodical Articles Related to Law*, University of Texas, 727 East 26th Street, Austin, TX 78705

(continued)

- *Inventory of Marriage and Family Literature (online and hard copy),* National Council on Family Relations, 3989 Central Avenue NE, Suite 550, Minneapolis, MN 55421

- *Mental Health Abstracts (online through DIALOG),* IFI/Plenum Data Company, 3202 Kirkwood Highway, Wilmington, DE 19808

- *PASCAL International Bibliography T205: Sciences de l'information Documentation,* INIST/CNRS-Service Gestion des Documents Primaires, 2, allee du Parc de Brabois, F-54514 Vandoeuvre-les-Nancy, Cedex, France

- *Periodical Abstracts, Research I* (general & basic reference indexing & abstracting data-base from University Microfilms International (UMI), 300 North Zeeb Road, P.O. Box 1346, Ann Arbor, MI 48106-1346), UMI Data Courier, P.O. Box 32770, Louisville, KY 40232-2770

- *Periodical Abstracts, Research II* (broad coverage indexing & abstracting data-base from University Microfilms International (UMI), 300 North Zeeb Road, P.O. Box 1346, Ann Arbor, MI 48106-1346), UMI Data Courier, P.O. Box 32770, Louisville, KY 40232-2770

- *Psychological Abstracts (PsycINFO),* American Psychological Association, P.O. Box 91600, Washington, DC 20090-1600

- *Sage Family Studies Abstracts (SFSA),* Sage Publications, Inc., 2455 Teller Road, Newbury Park, CA 91320

- *Social Work Abstracts,* National Association of Social Workers, 750 First Street NW, 8th Floor, Washington, DC 20002

- *Studies on Women Abstracts,* Carfax Publishing Company, P.O. Box 25, Abingdon, Oxfordshire OX14 3UE, United Kingdom

- *Violence and Abuse Abstracts: A Review of Current Literature on Interpersonal Violence (VAA),* Sage Publications, Inc., 2455 Teller Road, Newbury Park, CA 91320

- *Women Studies Abstracts,* Rush Publishing Company, P.O. Box 1, Rush, NY 14543

- *Women's Studies Index (indexed comprehensively),* G.K. Hall & Co., 866 Third Avenue, New York, NY 10022

(continued)

SPECIAL BIBLIOGRAPHIC NOTES

related to special journal issues (separates)
and indexing/abstracting

☐ indexing/abstracting services in this list will also cover material in any "separate" that is co-published simultaneously with Haworth's special thematic journal issue or DocuSerial. Indexing/abstracting usually covers material at the article/chapter level.

☐ monographic co-editions are intended for either non-subscribers or libraries which intend to purchase a second copy for their circulating collections.

☐ monographic co-editions are reported to all jobbers/wholesalers/approval plans. The source journal is listed as the "series" to assist the prevention of duplicate purchasing in the same manner utilized for books-in-series.

☐ to facilitate user/access services all indexing/abstracting services are encouraged to utilize the co-indexing entry note indicated at the bottom of the first page of each article/chapter/contribution.

☐ this is intended to assist a library user of any reference tool (whether print, electronic, online, or CD-ROM) to locate the monographic version if the library has purchased this version but not a subscription to the source journal.

☐ individual articles/chapters in any Haworth publication are also available through the Haworth Document Delivery Services (HDDS).

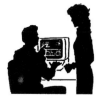

Women's Spirituality, Women's Lives

CONTENTS

ABOUT THE EDITORS

Judith Ochshorn, PhD, is Professor of Women's Studies at the University of South Florida where she co-founded the department more than twenty years ago and subsequently headed it for nine years. She teaches and publishes in the areas of women's history and feminist spirituality. Her book, *The Female Experience and the Nature of the Divine*, was submitted for a Pulitzer in Letters.

Ellen Cole, PhD, is a psychologist and sex therapist, and the Founding Dean of the Master of Arts Program at Prescott College in Arizona. She has recently moved to Anchorage, where she will be teaching in the Department of Psychology and Human Services, Alaska-Pacific University.

Introduction

Judith Ochshorn
Ellen Cole

More than twenty years ago a number of feminists, convinced that spirituality was central to human experience, charged Judaism and Christianity with betraying women. These feminists argued that the image of God as male in Jewish and Christian traditions legitimized male supremacy and female subordination on earth. The rule of the patriarch in heaven, celebrated in sexist symbols and metaphors, justified the rule of the fathers in the family and society.

Feminist spirituality is part of the current broad challenge to accepted ways of knowing and being. Like feminist accounts of the past, it is based on the critical insight that life experiences of women most often have differed from those of men, mediated, of course, by the influences of factors like class and ethnicity. Like feminist philosophy, it is exploring the significance of woman as "other," wrestling with the implications of the traditional view of the male, particularly the upper-class white male, as prototype of the human and the divine. Like feminist literary criticism, it is expanding our understanding of reality by viewing it through the eyes of the madwoman in the attic rather than exclusively through the rather ethnocentric lenses of Jane Eyre and Mr. Rochester. Like feminist psychology, it is reexamining what we mean by human nature and women's nature, re-valorizing and honoring those female traits that have been used to denigrate women and describe our inferiority.

[Haworth co-indexing entry note]: "Introduction." Ochshorn, Judith, and Ellen Cole. Co-published simultaneously in *Women & Therapy* (The Haworth Press, Inc.) Vol. 16, No. 2/3, 1995, pp. 1-4; and: *Women's Spirituality, Women's Lives* (ed: Judith Ochshorn, and Ellen Cole) The Haworth Press, Inc., 1995, pp. 1-4; and: *Women's Spirituality, Women's Lives* (ed: Judith Ochshorn, and Ellen Cole) Harrington Park Press, an imprint of The Haworth Press, Inc., 1995, pp. 1-4. Multiple copies of this article/chapter may be purchased from The Haworth Document Delivery Center [1-800-3-HAWORTH; 9:00 a.m. - 5:00 p.m. (EST)].

And underlying all of this has been the realization that our very understanding of reality—what comprises truth and knowledge, normalcy and virtue—depends on who defines it and what cultural baggage is brought to bear on that definition.

Emerging from these efforts and varying perspectives is a rich body of theories that collectively are redefining what it means to be a healthy woman and a healthy human being. But these theories move beyond the merely intellectual. Originating as they do in a profound sense of injustice, feminist theories are wedded to practice. They not only offer more accurate accounts of the past and critiques of the present than traditional theoretical perspectives but also point toward a transformed and far more humane future.

For those convinced of the importance of religion in women's lives, the 1970s was a heady time. While families tended to reserve serious study of the ways of God and man for males, the early, powerful voices raised against patriarchal aspects of Judaism and Christianity that legitimized such treatment resonated deeply, and laid the groundwork for present discussions. For example, Rosemary Radford Ruether exposed the connection of the mind/body split of ancient Greek and early Christian thought with gender hierarchy, and located her analyses in the context of class and race. Mary Daly argued that the mentality that makes God male and therefore sees maleness as godliness also is responsible for the triple horror, the "Unholy Trinity," of rape, genocide, and war. Carol Christ pointed out some of the compelling reasons why women need the Goddess. Judith Plaskow, in collaboration with other women, stood centuries of doctrine on its head by rewriting Genesis 2-3, basing her re-vision on the sisterhood of Eve and Lilith and joining the chorus that was reinterpreting original sin as sexism. And Starhawk and others were promoting alternatives like feminist wicca. While some abandoned religions altogether as hopelessly anti-woman, others staked out their own spiritual terrain and began to formulate a new ethic of connectedness not only to other women but to nature and the earth as well.

The 1980s saw a movement away from false universalism toward an emphasis on the importance of differences as well as commonalities among women and, therefore, a greater inclusiveness. Parallel to what transpired in every area of feminist analysis, the richness and range of a multiplicity of voices now incorporated under the aegis of feminist spirituality have resulted in efforts to speak to shared female experiences across the differences of class, race, ethnicity, sexual orientation, age, and physical abilities. Often in response to objections by women who felt marginalized by generalizations about gender that seemed to discount those differences by glossing over them, the conceptual parameters of feminist spirituality expanded in ways that enriched both feminist theories and the meanings of spirituality. While some reclaimed spiritual resources for themselves within existing religious traditions, others wove their own out of other cloth, and defined the sacred in their daily lives in new ways.

These days, there are women's groups in a variety of settings, from covens to women's caucuses to survivors' groups. While it's too early to tell about their enduring significance, we would argue (following the lead of Karen Brown) that we must attend not only to the stories women tell about their experiences but to the language participants in these groups use to describe them, e.g., words like "empowerment" and "healing." One might legitimately argue that there is no such thing as cheap grace, that, in fact, these groups in themselves cannot alter oppressive or alienating structures and beliefs and may, in fact, only produce what Marx referred to as false consciousness. Our illusions of power might only exacerbate our powerlessness. On the other hand, these women's groups may be necessary if not sufficient precursors of women's confrontations with society's oppressive structures and beliefs.

Across cultures, religious systems and the spiritual experiences they engendered have always provided one of the fundamental ways in which individuals and communities understand their relationships with each other, with their natural environments, and with whatever is believed to undergird those webs of relationships. They also have provided the means for individuals to express these understandings and the emotions they elicit through rituals. Together, they have provided a sense of rootedness and connectedness, a way for people to keep chaos at bay and feel some measure of control over their future.

To the extent that many kinds of women are beginning to assert our entitlement and capacity to identify, name, explore, and assess our own experiences, with the support and validation of other women, we may in fact be establishing that sense of rootedness and connectedness that religions have historically provided. Women are beginning to formulate new kinds of explanations about our relationships to other people, to nature, to what we see as the underlying sources of our lives congruent with our own rather than male experiences.

There are, of course, dangers. For example, traits like nurturance, that have been used to describe women's inferiority, may be indiscriminately valorized and may, in turn, create new narrow roads for female normalcy. Nevertheless, for all the possible pitfalls, and especially if we think of these developments as possible beginnings with difficult futures, we think the argument can be made that when we women tell our stories and, as Nelle Morton said, hear each other into speech, and when we create rituals that enable us to feel a sense of control over our future, we are moving not only toward establishing what has spiritual significance for us but also toward the kind of authority, agency, and autonomy that we associate with mental health and psychological well-being. The following essays explore some of the topography of that shift.

Shall We Gather at the River

Elizabeth Sargent

The night cracks open like a bottle
contents spilling
to every corner of the room
Poems slip through my fingers
wet as rain
even they can't save me
I ride the moon like a vampire
sucking the night away
I did it–I am the eye
that closes itself
when the dark grows red with weariness

There is nothing
that stares back at me
except the lit face of the clock
Each second is the footstep
in the hall   the hand
that twists the doorknob
the breath that burrows
in the smallest part of me

Elizabeth Sargent has an MA in English/Women's Studies. She is working towards a PhD in Women's Studies at the University of Oklahoma, and is a published poet.

This poem previously appeared in *Going Behind the Wall,* a chapbook published by Poetry Around Press, and is reprinted with permission of the author.

[Haworth co-indexing entry note]: "Shall We Gather at the River." Sargent, Elizabeth. Co-published simultaneously in *Women & Therapy* (The Haworth Press, Inc.) Vol. 16, No. 2/3, 1995, pp. 5-6; and: *Women's Spirituality, Women's Lives* (ed: Judith Ochshorn, and Ellen Cole) The Haworth Press, Inc., 1995, pp. 5-6; and: *Women's Spirituality, Women's Lives* (ed: Judith Ochshorn, and Ellen Cole) Harrington Park Press, an imprint of The Haworth Press, Inc., 1995, pp. 5-6.

Oh My sisters
shall we gather at the river
shall we sing Amazing Grace
Our scarred arms reach
for the lost mother
to come and wash our tired skin

Rosh Chodesh Dance
at the Summer Solstice

Janet Ruth Heller

The full moon rises,
But the sun stands still.
Now is the season
For dancing with women
On the hilltops
And in the valleys,
Around and around
In a sensuous circle
Embracing
All of my sisters
Until I feel
Whole again.

Janet Ruth Heller, PhD, teaches literature and creative writing at Grand Valley State University in Michigan. Her poetry has appeared in *Anima, Cottonwood Review, Organic Gardening, Women: A Journal of Liberation, Lilith, Modern Maturity, Mothers Today, The Writer, Our Mothers' Daughters, Women's Glib: A Collection of Women's Humor,* and *Modern Poems on the Bible: An Anthology.* She is a founding mother of *Primavera,* an award-winning women's literary magazine based in Chicago. Her book, *Coleridge, Lamb, Hazlitt, and the Reader of Drama,* was published in 1990 by the University of Missouri Press.

[Haworth co-indexing entry note]: "Rosh Chodesh Dance at the Summer Solstice." Heller, Janet Ruth. Co-published simultaneously in *Women & Therapy* (The Haworth Press, Inc.) Vol. 16, No. 2/3, 1995, p. 7; and: *Women's Spirituality, Women's Lives* (ed: Judith Ochshorn, and Ellen Cole) The Haworth Press, Inc., 1995, p. 7; and: *Women's Spirituality, Women's Lives* (ed: Judith Ochshorn, and Ellen Cole) Harrington Park Press, an imprint of The Haworth Press, Inc., 1995, p. 7. Multiple copies of this article/chapter may be purchased from The Haworth Document Delivery Center [1-800-3-HA-WORTH; 9:00 a.m. - 5:00 p.m. (EST)].

SECTION I:
LAYING THE GROUNDWORK

Women and Spirit:
Two Nonfits in Psychology

Mary Ballou

SUMMARY. The rules that guide the process of knowing in Western cultures are linked with the exclusion of certain realities. These rules of knowing shape what is known and are also linked with patriarchy, hierarchy, and oppression. Euro-American political, economic, and intellectual history forms a hegemony of interacting

Dr. Ballou is Associate Professor of Counseling Psychology at Northeastern University and a practicing psychologist in urban and rural areas. Her publications and clinical work reflect a variety of interests within Feminist Psychology.

Address correspondence to Department of Counseling Psychology, 203 Lake Hall, Northeastern University, 360 Huntington Avenue, Boston, MA 02115.

[Haworth co-indexing entry note]: "Women and Spirit: Two Nonfits in Psychology." Ballou, Mary. Co-published simultaneously in *Women & Therapy* (The Haworth Press, Inc.) Vol. 16, No. 2/3, 1995, pp. 9-20; and: *Women's Spirituality, Women's Lives* (ed: Judith Ochshorn, and Ellen Cole) The Haworth Press, Inc., 1995, pp. 9-20; and: *Women's Spirituality, Women's Lives* (ed: Judith Ochshorn, and Ellen Cole) Harrington Park Press, an imprint of The Haworth Press, Inc., 1995, pp. 9-20. Multiple copies of this article/chapter may be purchased from The Haworth Document Delivery Center [1-800-3-HAWORTH; 9:00 a.m. - 5:00 p.m. (EST)].

forces affecting the fabric of our lives and the nature and direction of our thoughts. This article, through the discussion of spirituality within psychology, explores the domination of certain ways of knowing and the necessity of including multiple epistemologies and multiple experiences within feminist psychology.

KNOWLEDGE, DEFINITION, AND CONTROL

The 17th century is historically key to the development of the rules for legitimate knowing: rationality and empiricism. Each of these has many earlier and later developments. But it is the 17th century which holds the victory of the secular claims of sensory observation and reason as the way to knowledge over the religious claims of knowledge by authority. The scientific method derives from 17th century assumptions about nature, universal laws, and how they may be known. The scientific revolution and the following enlightenment confirms the course of western intellectual and political development, and sets the agenda of patriarchy: material reality, science/logic, power/control. This agenda impacts upon contemporary western disciplines, intellectual and political world views, values, and cultural patterns. While it has allowed technological and economic development for *some*, unparalleled in recorded civilization, it has also encouraged disregard, unjust treatment and exclusion of many peoples and alternative ways of functioning and valuing and has devalued other modes of knowing. Accessing reality through direct experience, intuition, insight, connection with patterns, personal knowledge, and other experiential knowing modes is not considered legitimate within patriarchy's control of reality and its methods of knowledge generation.

Just as the narrow view of material reality and a controlling science restricts the methods of knowing, so too have they misunderstood and misevaluated indigenous cultural practices, values, and world views. These contentions have been amply discussed within the philosophy of science, feminist epistemology, feminist and liberation theology, interdisciplinary women's studies, African-Asian-Latin-Native American gender studies, critical analyses within traditional disciplines, and, to a lesser extent, in some feminist psychology.

MULTIPLE EPISTEMOLOGIES AND REALITY SHAPING

Epistemological methods and their shaping of reality have been discussed quite extensively and in several feminist literatures.[1] They point out that the method used to generate knowledge not only shows a different view of the phenomenon, but indeed shapes the phenomenon. Some examples illustrate the central points of the extensive and growing literature.

If we empirically seek to know about motivation by measuring observable behavior of performance in a laboratory, as McClelland did, then the reality of the phenomenon of motivation becomes competitive, physical actions, well tailored to capitalism. If, on the other hand, we ask activists what motivates them, we hear of commitment, principles, connections, standing with and against. Answers well fit for social change. In the first example, we see motivation as determined by the experimenter's assumptions, available measures, and prior *published* literature, which defines motivation as physical actions taken to achieve a desirable goal. In the second, real people living life and making choices tell us what urges and compels them to action. Reality is not only seen differently via each method of knowledge seeking, but the method shapes the reality. What a phenomenon is and how it is known are interactive.

A further illustration is the old Zen question: If a tree falls in the forest and no one is there to hear it, does it make a noise? Each epistemological method has a different answer or a different reason for the same answer. The empiricist says if it were not experienced by the senses, it is not real and, hence, no sound. So, too, would the phenomenologists say no, because it is outside their perceived experience. The rationalist and the nonrationalist would answer yes, there is a noise, yet for somewhat different reasons. The rationalist would, following the rules of logic, hold the tree's falling sound as a particular instance of general rules of mass striking mass with the resultant consequences described by physical laws of motion, mass, and sound. The nonrationalist would say yes as well, but because it

---

1. Included in the feminist discussions are: Harding (1986, 1992), Hartsock (1987), Keller (1985), Merchant (1980), Smith (1987), Weedon (1987), and Welch (1985), and in feminist psychology, Ballou (1990), Gergen (1988), Kaschak (1992), Riger (1992), and Unger (1988).

seems, feels, intuits so. Knowers by authority would look for the answer in Freud, their supervisor, the boss, or some other teacher, holy one, or prime source. Post-modernists would want to compile a discourse articulating the ontological status of treeing. Standpoint theorists would want to identify the categories of the judges in order to understand the gender, class, and culture shapings of the experience. Both would look to the social construction of the noise, trees, and forest.

Reason, empiricism/sensory experience, phenomenology/perceived knowledge, authority, and non-rational or intuition have all been identified as epistemological positions. Each of these has a valuable part to play in approaching reality. None is without limits. Each has particular strengths. Some may be better fitting for different kinds of reality seeking. However, none of the methods provide direct access to the truth of a phenomenon. Reality(ies) is (are) shaped by the method used to create/uncover/ engage it (them).

Reason and empiricism are at once familiar and thoroughly critiqued. Post-modern, phenomenology, and nonrational modes are less known and discussed. The standpoint and post-modern positions challenge the science/logic assumption of universal laws and basic truths. Post-modern analyses are important to ferreting out the contexts, exclusions, and subjectivity of knowledge claims. Knowing becomes relative and changing; a process. Post-modern theories can generate multiple views of spirituality with clarified contextual influences and subjugated stories.

Phenomenology and nonrational modes offer promising access to knowledge of spirituality. Phenomenology is quite appealing to some feminists, particularly as a method of research in the social science. Its strength is the placing of reality in experience and the mode of knowing in the perception of experience. Basing knowledge claims in actual lived experience is an effective way of generating knowledge because it requires careful attention to the actual experience, rather than imposing structure on that experience. It is especially useful in its attempt to gain cross cultural and other contextual understandings, and initial information ill-fitting to science/logic. It is limited, however, by the perceptual sets and processes of its user. If there is a particular schema, which there must be, then those structures shape the perceived experiences.

Since the view of dominant groups serves to blind its members to the equally valid, if different, views of less dominant groups, phenomenology's demand to place reality in actual experience is quite powerful. This is especially so when the category of difference is primary, as in cross cultural perception, where the goal is to understand the other's experience in their own terms and context. Listening to in order to hear the differences and commonalities is the task. Cross cultural spirit hunters often mistake or coopt the views of other cultures, relational and ontological attributes as a way to Truth, rather than as another example of the human urge for meaning and connection, and as a contextualized description of knowing.

Intuition, insight, and connection with patterns have often been wedded to a particular ideology about the universe and right living. However, as a method of knowing, nonrational modes may allow another access to experience, and one which may lead to a less controlled understanding of spirit. There are a number of descriptive phrases for this epistemological mode: knowing through direct experience or action; embodied knowledge which is a body sense inclusive of emotional and physical responses as arbitrators of knowledge; intuition; personal knowledge; connection with the transcendent (in feminist terms meaning across living beings rather than outside self); tactic knowledge; felt-sense, noetic experience; mystical; altered state of consciousness; enlightened knowing; christ/ buddha state; connection. It is a realm of experience to which there is little access from science/logic and patriarchy's ways of knowing and the traditional disciplines and languages which support them. It is, moreover, a kind of knowing which leads to a different understanding of spirituality. Some of the contemporary feminist and liberation theologies, wicca, earth, and ecological perspectives are participating in these phenomenological and nonrational modes of knowledge.

SPIRITUALITY

Much as woman-defined inclusion of women into psychology has confronted the theories, methods, and power arrangements within psychology, so too does the inclusion of spirituality confront views of reality and methods for coming to know it. Since most psychologists, psychiatrists, and social workers are trained in science and rationality and share in the privilege and perceptual set, looking at other modes of knowledge generation and their shaping of reality is difficult. It requires a suspension of fundamental assumptions and values in our thought, deeply ingrained by culture, Western history, professional socialization, and status hierarchy. This discussion of spirituality and women's psychology proceeds against such a background of linkages between epistemologies, realities, and power relations. Spirituality is a dimension of human experience, a reality experienced through specific modes of knowing. For some it is a lens through which to view one's own and others' existence. Western intellectual traditions neither validate this reality nor legitimize epistemological methods to access the dimension of spirituality. Those wanting to explore spirituality, feeling the need for additional qualities of meaning, or pulled to experience life as mattering, have had to look to religious traditions, counterculture principled movements, or sensibilities, rituals, and beliefs originally described in other cultures' traditions.

Traditional views of spirituality have been shaped by the patriarchy to make the spiritual become separate, beyond natural, and arranged in hierarchical relationships. There are holy men and mystics who are certainly different from us.

There are Buddhist priests who attain insight, transcend ordinary life, and become teachers. Those who know about or are spiritual are special, better than, and separate. Evolved spirituality is a higher developmental stage won by very few. They achieve individuation and separation of self from their supportive environments. Patriarchal culture uses its norms to shape the traditional views of spirituality, to institutionalize it, to make experts and controllers.

Spirituality, distinct from this patriarchal misshaping, is within our ordinary life experiences, states of consciousness, relationships with others, attunements with nature and life patterns, and states of being. Some indigenous world views offer glimpses of spiritual views. Some are: harmony with the rhythms of nature in North American Native peoples; the nonmaterial richness of some Asian cultures; the noncomplex peace, work, prayer of monastic Christians; the community identities of some African Americans. These experiences in so far as we understand them connect with our intuition and compel attention. The stories, rituals and world views hold descriptions of knowing through nonrational modes and experience. Cultural beliefs and traditions and various value and religious narratives stand as evidence of the human need/capacity for spirituality.

Feminist views of spirituality offer importantly different views, ones which encourage us to reflect upon our own lives, relationships, actions, our felt connection experiences and our meaning making. For instance, Ochs (1989) writes about a feminist view of spirituality which is natural, readily available, and surrounding us all.

> Spirituality is a process of coming into relationship with reality. It is a process of not just knowing but a way of being and doing. A process of connecting with what is real. We experience and reflect on our experience, but more than that, we have a relationship to our experiences and reflections. The active, conscious, deliberate process of coming into this relationship is the beginning of spirituality. (pp. 9-10)

Feminist spirituality is placed in ordinary life, is known through experience, and holds relationship central. Ochs describes coming into relationship with the reality of one's own experiences, Harrison (1989) with just actions, Heyward (1993) with mutual connections amongst other people, Williams (1989) with relationship in community, Spretnak (1991) with the earth, and Sanchez (1993) with the land, the tribe, and the natural rhythms. While each of these women develops her own reflections on one or several aspects of connectedness, the grounding in relationship and connection is unmistakable.

Feminist theology is based in the multiple and diverse experiences of women with careful attention to and reflection on those experiences. It is available to all and authored from one's own felt sense and connections. The call to action for earth healing, restoration of natural patterns, mutual relational engagement, equitable resources, liberation from domination in person, politic and mind, and recognizing and accepting difference as equally valid, is a powerful project–a project with multiple modes of knowing.

Spirituality may be characterized as a specific consciousness, resultant from reflection on one's own lived/felt experience, as connected to and in relationship with self, others, and communities. The particular consciousness may be facilitated by symbols, rituals, actions, and focused attending. In this sense spirituality is a level of perception readily available to us. An aspect of experience, grounded in life affirming and in this state, self-evident, principles which impel us to connection with and action for others. Spirituality may be described as a process of knowing and relating rather than a particular content. Spirituality may be a way of perceiving the intrinsic within distinctive states of consciousness. Knowing through access to felt experience and reflection may be essential to this perceptual shift. This knowing leads to experiencing relationship with, and being connected to, in multiple dimensions.

Spirituality, while nonsense and nonrational to Western science/logic, is a natural part of human experience. It is accessible to those who choose to realize their felt experience and who dare to risk awareness and exploration of phenomena which are denied or marginalized in dominant Euro-American culture. Traditional and certainly academic psychology have not and can not attend to spirituality. Spirit is a problematic reality and it requires a problematic mode of knowing for psychology, because traditional psychology does not have a diversity of modes of knowing. Science of behavior requires material realities known through sensory experience and their logical extensions. Spirituality requires modes of knowing and conceptions of realities which are far more diverse.

THE PROMISE AND CONSTRAINT
OF RECENT FEMINIST PSYCHOLOGY

Some of the work within the Psychology of Women has developed beyond the science/logic participation of psychology in its attention to gender within psychology. Yet much is still based only in and constrained by the patriarchy's knowing modes. Feminism has become a system of analysis, in addition to a set of values and commitments. It is approaching paradigm status as the assumptions, methods, rules, and relationship between these and the questions asked expand. Multiple modes of knowing and exploration of realities beyond those shaped by and appropriate for science/logic are also entering into psychology's feminism.

Newly heard theories and clinical practices based in women's experiences, reexamination of power distributions in relationships and practices, equally valued differences, and multi-influenced (including the socio-political) sources of damage and development are important. Some of these efforts are nearing the spiritual domain. The theory building based in relationship and growthful, healing connections of the Stone Center's self-in-relation is one of several examples. Within the general community of developing theory and practice, Judith Jordan's work on empathy (1990, 1991) seems particularly coalescing. She makes empathy feminist. Beyond understanding and appreciating another's world as Carl Rogers held, she sees empathy as an experience of mutual connection. In distinction to empathy as a necessary condition for separated self growth toward a goal of fully functioning, she holds empathic connection as the essence of healing. Jordan has come to stress the process of mutual connection, two women connecting with each other, thus redistributing the power and basing the process in experience. This in contrast to the kind and sympathetic expert who through rational analysis buttressed by science will treat the patient's illness.

While Judith Jordan does not use the word "spiritual," the mutual empathic connection of which she writes participates in the spiritual domain. Is the heresy of spirit to science/material logic constraining the use of the word in "serious scholarship"? Moreover the reliance of self-in-relation theory on revised psychodynamic and especially object relations theory for validation places the theory in rationality which can not handle spirituality or intuitional knowing. Women's experiences and reflection on them may well be the source of the insights, yet rational analysis via logic and authorities in mainstream personality theory are the supporting references. It seems that the self-in-relation model will continue to be constrained until the epistemology of experience becomes a main, rather than a ghost, author. Only then will spirituality within connection not sound so alien and be so heretical to psychology's scholarship tradition.

. Another example within feminist psychology offers an illustration of the value of reflection on diverse experiences. Judith Herman's work on trauma (1992), with the addition of Maria Root's

(1992) broader conceptualization, is an important illustration because it demonstrates the knowledge gained from race experience and reflection. The addition of Root's model of trauma to that of Herman's yields a richer and more responsive conceptualization of trauma. Class, race, and culture are considered in the causes and damaging effects of trauma. A fuller response to diverse and contextualized model building offered by Root enhances Herman's notions of trauma. For instance, Root brings conceptions of "indirect" and "insidious" to the views of trauma. Insidious and indirect trauma, neglected in most of the trauma literature, stem from central consideration of the varieties of life conditions amongst peoples and the multiple forms of oppression and subtle experiences. Similarly Root's consideration of intent (malicious or accidental) and context (isolation or companion) and finally the integration of the earlier crisis literature makes her model of trauma richer and more connected to an older literature and to oppression beyond gender. Root brings astute and more responsive model building to the joining. Yet Herman's work in the stages of treatment and their interactive nature is immensely important. In particular, her attention to the importance of community in the third phase of recovery legitimizes alternative modes of treatment and healing. Or turned around, individual remediative psychotherapy is educated and strengthened by strategies of community support and healing. Also, by presenting (and here she is describing her reflections of experience) the importance of community, Herman invites consideration of the defining and healing power of connection beyond self and therapist. She opens the door to further exploration and description of relationship, action and healing phenomena central to feminist conceptions of spirituality. Root and Herman's work together offers much to feminist psychology. If community, spirit healing, and social change strategies, there for the gifting by "the others," were added, feminist psychology and mental health would be a fine creation.

Powerful guides in the development of feminist psychologies result from the linkages of epistemologies, control of knowing, patriarchy, and spirituality. Carefully describing and reflecting upon relationships, social/political structures and meaning and valuing of nondominant groups, as well as multiple modes of knowing, hold promise for development in unconstrained directions. Reexamining ideas from intuition and experience extends and holds promise to transform traditional notions. Women's experiences, epistemologies, the spirit as process and content, and their connections are all central to the continuing development of feminist psychology. Feminist Psychology must refuse the hegemony of patriarchic control within our discipline and within our theory and practice. The politics of exclusion must be disempowered in our focus, our content, and our knowing structures.

REFERENCES

Adams, C. (Ed.). (1993). *Ecofeminism and the sacred*. New York: Continuum Publishing.

Ballou, M. (1990). Approaching a feminist-principled paradigm in the construction of personality theory. In Brown, L. & Root M. *Diversity and complexity in feminist therapy*. New York: The Haworth Press, Inc.

Gergen, M. (Ed.). (1988). *Feminist thought and the structure of knowledge*. New York: New York University Press.

Harding, S. (1991). *Whose science? Whose knowledge?* Ithaca, NY: Cornell University Press.

Harding, S. (1986). *The science question in feminism*. Ithaca, NY: Cornell University Press.

Harrison, B. (1989). The Power of anger in the work of love. In J. Plaskow & C. Christ (Eds.) *Weaving the vision*. San Francisco: Harper Collins.

Hartsock, N. (1987). The Feminist standpoint: Developing the ground for a specifically feminist materialism. In Harding (Ed.) *Feminism & methodology*. Bloomington: Indiana University Press.

Herman, J. (1992). *Trauma and recovery*. New York: Basic Books.

Heyward, C. (1993). *When boundaries betray us*. San Francisco: Harper Collins.

Jordan, J., Kaplan, A., Miller, J., Stiver, I., & Surrey, J. (1991). *Women's growth in connection*. New York: Guilford.

Jordan, J. (1990). Courage in connection. *Work in Progress* #29. Wellesley , MA: Stone Center Working Papers.

Kaschak, E. (1992). *Engendered lives*. New York: Basic Books.

Keller, E. (1985). *Reflections on science and gender*. New Haven: Yale University Press.

Merchant, C. (1980). *The death of nature*. San Francisco: Harper & Row.

Ochs, C. (1989). *Women and spirituality*. Totowa, NJ: Rowman & Allanheld.

Riger, S. (1992). Epistemological debates, feminist voices: science, social values and the study of women. *American Psychologist*. 47, 730-740.

Root, M. (1992). Reconstructing the impact of trauma on personality. In L. Brown, & M. Ballou (Eds.) *Personality and psychopathology*. NY: Guilford.

Sanchez, C. (1993). Animal, vegetable, and mineral. In C. Adams (Ed.) *Ecofeminism and the sacred*. NY: Continuum.

Smith D. (1987). Women's perspective as radical critique of sociology. In Harding (3d) *Feminism & methodology*. Bloomington: Indiana University Press.

Spretnak, C. (1991). *States of grace*. San Francisco: Harper Collins.

Unger, R. (1988). Psychology, feminist and personal epistemology. In M. Gergen (Ed.) *Feminist thoughts and the structure of knowledge*. NY: New York University Press.

Weedon, C. (1987). *Feminist practice & poststructuralist theory*. NY: Basil Blackwell.

Welch, S. (1985). *Communities of resistance and solidarity*. Maryknoll, N.Y.: Orbis Books.

Williams, D. (1989). Womanist theology. In Plaskow & Christ. *Weaving the vision*. San Francisco: Harper Collins.

Psychological Implications
of Women's Spiritual Health

Mary E. Hunt

SUMMARY. The burgeoning women's spirituality movement is concrete evidence of feminist awakening in the culture. Women are finding some forms of feminist spirituality helpful for good mental health. Three specific shifts which have been occasioned by the feministization of religion are: (1) Women as protagonists of religion; (2) Women role models in the ministry, the academic study of religion, and as healers and leaders; and (3) Feminist changes in the content of the world's religions. This feminist theological overview clarifies the dynamics so that mental health professionals will understand what is happening and how it might figure into their strategies for health and healing.

INTRODUCTION

Psychology and religion have been uneasy partners at best in patriarchal cultures. They have competed for intellectual and spiritual hegemony, each insisting that it has the final word on health. Feminist work in both fields is beginning to change that dynamic

---

Mary E. Hunt, PhD, is a feminist theologian, currently Co-Director of the Women's Alliance for Theology, Ethics and Ritual (WATER), 8035 13th Street, Silver Spring, MD. Her many publications include *Fierce Tenderness: A Feminist Theology of Friendship*, for which she won the Crossroad Women's Studies Prize.

[Haworth co-indexing entry note]: "Psychological Implications of Women's Spiritual Health." Hunt, Mary E. Co-published simultaneously in *Women & Therapy* (The Haworth Press, Inc.) Vol. 16, No. 2/3, 1995, pp. 21-32; and: *Women's Spirituality, Women's Lives* (ed: Judith Ochshorn, and Ellen Cole) The Haworth Press, Inc., 1995, pp. 21-32; and: *Women's Spirituality, Women's Lives* (ed: Judith Ochshorn, and Ellen Cole) Harrington Park Press, an imprint of The Haworth Press, Inc., 1995, pp. 21-32. Multiple copies of this article/chapter may be purchased from The Haworth Document Delivery Center [1-800-3-HAWORTH; 9:00 a.m. - 5:00 p.m. (EST)].

21

mutual recognition of the interdisciplinary approach necessary to do our respective jobs (Goldenberg, 1990; Randour, 1987).

Contemporary feminist theologians are deeply indebted to the social sciences as renewed by feminists scholars in the various fields for insights and input into the human condition which are now being crafted with women's well being as central. Feminist psychological professionals are beginning to explore the implications of the "feministization" of religion, learning as they go that many women are finding in women's spiritual groups elements of health and healing that they seek. By feministization I mean the process by which the needs and experiences of those previously marginalized, especially women, but including others such as those who are economically poor and racially discriminated against, are taken as normative in the shaping of religion.

The burgeoning women's spirituality movement is a concrete manifestation of the feminist awakening in the culture. Thirty years ago a search for gender-specific women's groups would have yielded the Altar and Rosary Society, a women's circle or guild of a small church, or perhaps a charitable arm of a congregation. In the late twentieth century, virtually every major religious tradition has felt the impact of this process. New religious forms have sprung up, ancient religious practices have been revitalized, and some women are simply claiming for themselves a religious dimension to their lives without regard for connection to a specific tradition.

As a feminist theologian, indeed as a Euro-American of Roman Catholic heritage who participates in the women-church movement and actively dismantles hierarchical Catholicism whenever possible, I understand and appreciate the deep suspicion which many psychological professionals have harbored about patriarchal religions. Most feminist theologians share this suspicion since we have seen up close the damage which has been done to people and the earth in the name of the divine. We abhor and seek to eradicate the patronizing and duplicitous behavior used by some religious professionals to maintain structures of dominance. Many of us have experienced the damage which has been done to women, always the majority of a religious group, who have had little if any influence in its shaping, and who have had a great deal of power exerted over them by those traditions.

At the same time, feminist theologians respect religious search for those who choose it, and seek to assure the human right to religious integrity, that is, to the wholeness religious people claim. This does not mean that everyone need be religious, rather that those who wish to be can find ways that are liberating and not oppressive, involving of them rather than imposed upon them. Feminist work in religion, what I call the feministization of religion, is aimed at doing just that.

The process of undoing and/or redoing centuries of tradition is slow. Psychological professionals know that from the difficulty of undoing Freudian and Jungian "gospels" which are of far more recent vintage than most of their religious counterparts. As the work of feminist theology progresses, there is growing evidence that women are finding some forms of feminist spirituality helpful rather than harmful. I submit that further exploration is warranted in order to assure that mental health professionals understand what is happening and how it might figure into their strategies for health and healing.

Even if we were to disagree on the relative importance of our respective fields, the conversations among us can go on in realistic ways based on feminist work and not on an outmoded notion of what is normative in our fields. Just as male constructed psychologies are giving way to feminist critiques, so too are paradigms shifting in religion, remarkable as it may seem.

In this essay I will outline the changes from the perspective of a feminist theologian. For reasons of brevity, I will confine most of my analysis to the Christian context though it is important to note that similar dynamics are at work in other traditions as well. I will provide a brief overview of the religious scene, then explore three specific shifts which I think have been occasioned by the feministization of religion insofar as they have an impact on women: (1) Women as protagonists of religion; (2) Women role models in the ministry, the academic study of religion, and as healers and leaders; and (3) Feminist changes in the content of the world's religions.

I will conclude with several observations of their implications for good mental health. I hope that this will serve as an invitation to therapists to consider probing religious issues with their clients with a new openness to the possibility that feminist religions might play a constructive part despite their dismal patriarchal past.

THE "FEMINISTIZATION" OF RELIGION

The late twentieth century is distinguished by the proliferation of women's work in religion. Lest I seem unduly enthusiastic about relatively small progress, it should be noted that this stands in contrast to centuries of almost nothing, hence inflating the extent of the work rather than signaling quantum leaps. It is beyond the scope of this essay to catalogue all of the advances, but a sample will suffice to show the degree to which this work has permeated the field.

Feminist theology parallels feminist theory in its deconstruction and reconstruction of concepts, practices and structures which heretofore have passed over women and women's experiences. Feminist theology is but one source, predicated largely on the experiences of Euro-American women. Womanist work based on the experiences of African American women, mujerista based on the experiences of Hispanic women, and Asian women's theologies all shape the contours of this effort (Isasi-Diaz, 1993; Kung, 1990; Williams, 1993). Each of these has its own methodology and priorities. As a feminist I am indebted to them but in no way represent them. A reflection such as this one from each of those starting points is necessary to round out the analysis since gender, race, class, sexual integrity, age, national origin, etc., are interdependent variables in the feministization process. My effort here simply starts the process.

In the United States, explicit attention to women's concerns can be traced to the late nineteenth century when suffrage leaders like Elizabeth Cady Stanton and colleagues took on the immodest but typically feminist task of revising the Bible using women's experiences as normative (Stanton, 1895/1974). Their insight, that society would not change without concomitant changes in religion, continues to guide the theo-political work feminist theologians do today. One hundred years later, biblical scholars have shown that interpretations were deliberately skewed to favor masculinist biases and that women were systematically written out of Christian history beginning with the scriptures (Schussler Fiorenza, 1993).

Mary Daly opened the Pandora's box of religion when she claimed that "if God is male, then the male is God" (Daly, 1973, p. 19). The twenty years since her claim have seen unprecedented strides toward dismantling patriarchal structures and replacing them with inclusive ones, a process which is still in its infancy. More to our point, Mary Daly's invitation to move "beyond God the Father" was just the intellectual permission many people needed to exit patriarchal religions and discover that the sky would not fall in, that life would go on with much increased autonomy.

Nearly every nook and cranny of Christian theology has been up-ended by feminist work. Revised historical materials have emerged showing previously hidden contributions of women. Theological language and imagery–including such previously sacrosanct notions of Lord, Father, Ruler and King–have changed such that now inclusivity is increasingly common, though by no means normative, in hymns, prayers and sermons. The entrance of large numbers of women into the ministry is rapidly changing what was previously an all male arena. Predictions are that the field will become, like nursing and teaching, largely female due to the long hours, relatively low pay, constant availability and endless nurture which add up to a recipe for a female job in a patriarchal society.

Some of the most obvious changes are taking place in the arena of theological ethics, especially issues of reproductive health and lifestyle, where women's input was previously unknown. Likewise, in liturgy and ritual, there is beginning to appear in even the most mainstream churches some hint that pulpit-down-to-people sermons and hocus-pocus sacraments by mumbling priests are simply inadequate to the spiritual needs and demands of religious adherents.

I call this process "feministization" to distinguish it from "feminization," that is, from efforts to lift up women's ways of being religious, what is often referred to as a "women and" approach, as if some essential female elements could be discerned. That approach only reinforces gender stereotypes in patriarchy and does not address the complexity of interlocking oppressions nor power differentials. Feminism, by contrast, takes for granted that gender is but one of many interconnected categories which form a tight web of oppression. For example, women of so-called minority racial ethnic groups experience oppression differently, that is, to a degree that is multiplied by their oppressions, than Euro-American women; lesbian women experience it differently than heterosexual women, and so forth. Analyses of these differences and the differences they make characterize feminist work (Schussler Fiorenza, 1992, p. 114).

Patriarchy is not simply a religious concept, but a secular one in which power is stratified and concentrated in the hands of a few throughout society. Religions in patriarchy shore up the system by providing its theological underpinnings, literally baptizing and confirming notions of dominance with religious ideology. Feminist theological work undercuts the foundations by challenging the hegemony of dominant categories and replacing the pyramidal model with circles. Needless to say this work takes its toll on feminists who are a correctly perceived threat to the religious status quo. We mean to disrupt its damaging impact on individuals and societies, and we interpret the backlash against us as a measure of our success.

Similar efforts are taking place in virtually all religious traditions with varying results. The phenomenon in Christian churches is not limited to the United States, but is found all over the world, from women's base communities in Argentina to the World Council of Churches' Decade of Churches in Solidarity with Women, from religiously inspired efforts to eradicate violence in the Philippines to efforts toward Roman Catholic women's ordination to the priesthood in Bangladesh, not to mention the myriad groups which meet privately for their own edification.

Jewish feminists are making enormous strides in reconceptualizing their tradition (Plaskow, 1990). Buddhist women are equally energetic in their efforts (Gross, 1993). Hindu and Muslim women are bringing their traditions into dialogue with contemporary feminist thought (Teays, 1991; Mernissi, 1985). Some of the most far-reaching efforts are in Wicca, Goddess worship, women's spirit and Gaia which do not have to contend with the stonewalling of entrenched authorities (Gimbutas, 1989; Starhawk, 1979, 1989).

This sketch, albeit partial, suggests that just as the world will never be the same after feminism, neither will the world's religions. What does this mean in terms of women's mental and spiritual health?

WOMEN'S SPIRITUALITY
IN THE WAKE OF PATRIARCHY

I do not mean to paint too rosy a picture of women's religiosity in light of the backlash against feminism, and the backlash against backlash, or whiplash, which makes it difficult to know just how to overcome certain problems. For example, the ordination of women in the Roman Catholic Church is increasingly likely. But to ordain women into hierarchical structures and de facto demand that they be celibate and under the direct control of male bishops will be no great accomplishment. It will undoubtedly shore up hierarchical church structures, reinforce the most oppressive aspects of the tradition, and leave untouched the many doctrinal and dogmatic issues which are so problematic. Thus it is crucial that we not confuse unhealthy traps set in patriarchy to coopt women with healthy efforts to empower women.

Nonetheless, the proliferation of women's spiritual groups such as women-church, Goddess, women-spirit and other brands around the country leads me to suggest that enormous changes are taking place. I cluster these advances as they affect psychology in three areas:

1. Women as Protagonists of Religion

The major change in the feministization of religion is not in the gender of the divine, though female imagery and symbolism, as well as more abstract, non-gendered notions are important. Rather it is the idea that women are not meant to be passive recipients of religion but active shapers, what Latin American women have called agents or protagonists of religion. This signals a fundamental change from a hierarchical model with religious professionals whether female or male in charge to women taking responsibility for our own religious lives. It means not clericalizing women but declericalizing churches, for example, structuring women's worship groups without leaders and followers but with rotating leadership. It means replacing what I think of as a "Jeopardy" model of doing theology in which answers are given to questions we did not ask, with an invitation to women to ask and answer our own questions of ultimate meaning and value.

I repeat that this is not popular among patriarchal religious officials, and is perceived correctly to be a threat to mainline religions, but it is increasingly characteristic of feminist religious efforts. For example, the women-church movement is a network of feminist base communities which gather in the homes of members for worship, informal sharing and strategizing for social change. Many of the groups in the U.S. are made up of women who have long since left patriarchal Christianity, especially Catholicism, preferring to fashion their own ways of *being* church rather than simply struggling to change their churches. Ignoring power structures, in this case churches, and especially withholding financial support, hastens their demise.

This is evidence of healthy religiosity which I believe is to be encouraged. Far from being the "opiate of the people," I submit that women coming together around religious themes, whether for worship, discussion and/or social action can be very positive. Of course such groups often develop their own problems and their own pathological dynamics. Their content requires critical appraisal as well. But my observation is that normally they are places where women find nurture and support, where it is safe to ask questions and share ideas, where they can act out convictions and explore spirituality.

Many such groups meet regularly for a meal, time for checking in and discussing members' personal lives, as well as whatever explicitly religious content they share. This can lead to the formation of strong commitments unto a sense of community for the members. I see this as helpful in a patriarchal society which would atomize and isolate women. But the key point is that women are in charge, women make choices and empower others to do the same, and women use their collective energy for social change.

From a mental health perspective this means that women increase their opportunities for collective autonomy from one more patriarchal institution, namely, religion. Women practice naming and claiming their own issues and beliefs. They create liturgies and rituals which reflect their deepest experiences, for example, first menstruation, coming out as a lesbian, entering menopause, hardly the stuff of Sunday services in patriarchal religions (Neu, 1991, 1993). Further, such groups provide a place to articulate feelings with the expectation that these will be taken seriously, as well as opportunities to grapple with ultimate meaning and value in the development of religious ethics.

I do not pretend that such groups are always helpful, but I note that they are qualitatively different from patriarchal religions in the fact that women are unabashedly in charge. Some few of the groups include male participants, but even in those instances the fact that women are protagonists and not bystanders in the shaping of the religious ideology makes a world of difference.

2. Women Role Models in the Ministry, the Academic Study of Religion, and as Healers and Leaders

Another result of the feministization of religion is the creation of role models. When I began theological studies in the late 1960s there simply were not any women role models aside from a handful of theologically trained nuns whose lifestyle, frankly, did not attract me. Now young women can see that it is possible to be a rabbi, priest, minister or bishop, albeit usually on patriarchal terms, but always with the possibility of transforming the model.

While it is still hard to transform these roles within the confines of patriarchy, happily there are women in religion who do so, often at great personal cost. These women function as helpful professionals in those liminal moments when one might turn to religion for support, for example, on the death of a parent or partner, or in the event of a covenant or marriage. While therapeutic help is often beneficial, many people also need and want to deal with such matters in the public forum, or, in the case of marriage, must do so because of legal requirements. Further, many people want to explore a spiritual dimension, for instance, during illness or when seeking meaning in life itself. It need not be done, but for those who wish to do so, feminist religious accompaniment is something I trust over the patriarchal option.

Women theologians provide a great deal of mentoring for younger women in the field. Whereas "feminist" is still a dirty word in certain academic circles, and gender studies in religion are blunting some of the sharper analytic edges, it is apparent that successive generations of feminist scholars are making an impact. Mainline seminaries are virtually forced to include feminist work on their bibliographies and among course offerings. Even those who reject it are prodded as a matter of professional standards to be conversant with it. It is obvious at guild meetings such as the American Academy of Religion or the Society for Biblical Literature, which have segments on Women and Religion, Lesbian Issues in Religion, Womanist Approaches to Religion and Society, Feminist Theory and Theology, Women in the Biblical World and so forth, that some of the most creative work is emerging in these settings.

Likewise, women religious leaders, though fewer in number, are having an impact. Whether it be Mama Lola, a Haitian Vodou priestess, or Bishop Barbara Harris, the first woman bishop of the Episcopal Church, young people are seeing women as religious leaders as never before (Brown, 1991).

Mental health workers, I suggest, should note this as another example of women's empowerment. I predict that while most of these role models are still enmeshed in patriarchal contexts, over time there will be discernable progress toward feminist models of ministry, academic collaboration and religious leadership. Meanwhile, the benefits of such role models for sparking others to attempt similar work far outweigh my reservations.

3. Feminist Changes in the Content of the World's Religions

Women's entrance into the world's religions in unprecedented numbers and with unapologetic agency has meant substantive changes in religious content. The most obvious examples are inclusive language and imagery which signal theological shifts. For instance, God as mother or friend is substantially different from God as father, though I would encourage people to ask why god at all. But the point is that we are no longer content with cosmetic changes, and are probing well beneath the surface. For example, in Christian theology feminists are not asking whether Jesus was a feminist, rather what kind of a god would give up "his" only begotten son even for so lofty a purpose as the supposed salvation of the world. It is hard to imagine a mother, god or otherwise, who would consider such an action (Brown & Parker, 1989). This direct challenge to the long-standing Christian doctrine of the atonement is an example of the depth of feminist critique.

Violence is now a prominent theological concern. We are probing whether and how religious traditions exacerbate violence rather than eradicate it. We are concerned with the religious images and symbols which, however implicitly, sanction violence, for example the wrath of God. There is no question but that the content that results from such scrutiny will be different. The question is how or whether what remains and/or is constructed is part of the same tradition. For example, is Christianity without the cross still Christianity? Many of us do not care, preferring instead our religious commitment to be expressed in the eradication of violence rather than in the preservation of a specific religious tradition. That shift in focus marks a real change.

For those who concern themselves with religion from a mental health stand point it is important to know that one result of the feministization of religion is new content. While I make no claims about our having solved perennial problems, I do believe that we are opening up the process of religious development so that the experiences of more people will shape the outcome. Hopefully, the process itself will remain dynamic and open-ended rather than static and truncated. At least this is the challenge we have set for ourselves and are pursuing as we move into the twenty-first century as feminist religious professionals.

CONCLUSION

The feministization of religion is just beginning. But already we have seen increased collective autonomy and renewed opportunities for women to express and find support. We have seen an increase in role models both among religious professionals and academics. And, we are seeing substantive rather than simply cosmetic changes in the content of the world's religions.

I can imagine some mental health professionals arguing that the same projections and myths of religion are simply being dressed in women's clothing. But I think that is to miss the fundamental point, namely, that in patriarchy clothing is gender coded, but that feministization means that we can wear what is comfortable, what fits well and what catches our fancy. Now we can try on the religious robes of our choosing, or choose to go without, and expect that our choices will be increasingly feasible, available, economical, and above all, respected. They will not cover or make up for the problems of the past, but they will gird us for the possibilities of a feminist religious future. That alone is reason enough to pay attention to them, and encouragement enough to consider them healthy.

REFERENCES

Brown, Joanne C. & Parker, Rebecca. (1989). For God so loved the world? In Joanne C. Brown & Carole R. Bohn (Eds.), *Christianity, patriarchy and abuse: A feminist critique* (pp. 1-30). New York: The Pilgrim Press.

Brown, Karen M. (1991). *Mama lola: A vodou priestess in Brooklyn.* Berkeley: University of California Press.

Daly, Mary. (1973). *Beyond God the father.* Boston: Beacon Press.

Gimbutas, Marija. (1989). *The language of the goddess.* San Francisco: Harper and Row.

Goldenberg, Naomi R. (1990). *Returning words to flesh: Feminism, psychoanalysis, and the resurrection of the body.* Boston: Beacon Press.

Gross, Rita M. (1993). *Buddhism after patriarchy.* Albany, NY: State University of New York Press.

Isasi-Diaz, Ada Maria. (1993). *En la lucha: A hispanic women's liberation theology.* Minneapolis: Fortress Press.

Kung, Chung Hyun. (1990). *Struggle to be the sun again: Introducing asian women's theology.* Maryknoll, NY: Orbis Books.

Mernissi, Fatima. (1985). *Beyond the veil: Male-female dynamics in modern muslim society.* Cambridge, MA: Schenkman Publishing Co.

Neu, Diann L. (1991). Choosing wisdom: A croning ceremony. *WATERwheel, 6*(3), 4-5.

Neu, Diann L. (1993). We are all daughters: Healing the daughter/mother relationship. *WATERwheel, 6*(1), 4-5.

Plaskow, Judith. (1990). *Standing again at sinai: Judaism from a feminist perspective.* San Francisco: Harper and Row.

Randour, Mary Lou. (1987). *Women's psyche, women's spirit: The reality of relationships.* New York: Columbia University Press.

Schussler Fiorenza, Elisabeth. (1992). *But she said.* Boston: Beacon Press.

Stanton, Elizabeth C. & the Revising Committee. (1974). *The woman's bible.* Seattle, WA: Coalition Task Force on Women and Religion. (Original work published 1895).

Starhawk. (1989). *The spiral dance: A rebirth of the ancient religion of the great goddess.* (rev. ed.) San Francisco: Harper and Row.

Teays, Wanda. (1991). The burning bride: The dowry problem in India. *Journal of Feminist Studies in Religion, 7*(2), 29-52.

Williams, Delores S. (1993). *Sisters in the wilderness: The challenge of womanist god-talk.* Maryknoll, NY: Orbis Books.

Feminist Metanoia and Soul-Making

Rosemary Radford Ruether

SUMMARY. This article critiques the traditional Christian under-standing of sin and alienation and the process of conversion through reception of transcendent grace. It reconstructs the understanding of human transformation from a perspective of feminist spirituality and ethics. Fallenness is reenvisioned in terms of women's subjugation by patriarchal social and cultural systems, and conversion is seen in terms of the process by which women's journey leads them to ques-tion these systems and embark on a process of emancipation from them to create a new self and a new society. Both alienation and transformation are viewed in terms of the interrelation of the psychic and the social.

In this article I will explore feminist metanoia and soul-making. I will speak of feminism, not simply as political analysis and social change, although it is surely that, but how feminism calls both women and men into personal and social conversion and trans-formation. Let me begin by saying something about how I under-

Rosemary Radford Ruether holds MA and PhD degrees from the Claremont Graduate School in Claremont, California in Classics and Early Christian History. She is presently the Georgia Harkness Professor of Applied Theology at the Garrett Theological Seminary and a member of the graduate faculty of North-western University, 2121 Sheridan Road, Evanston, IL 60201.
This essay was originally given as a plenary address at the annual meeting of the Association of Clinical-Pastoral Counselers.

[Haworth co-indexing entry note]: "Feminist Metanoia and Soul-Making." Ruether, Rosemary Radford. Co-published simultaneously in *Women & Therapy* (The Haworth Press, Inc.) Vol. 16, No. 2/3, 1995, pp. 33-44; and: *Women's Spirituality, Women's Lives* (ed: Judith Ochshorn, and Ellen Cole) The Haworth Press, Inc., 1995, pp. 33-44; and: *Women's Spirituality, Women's Lives* (ed: Judith Ochshorn, and Ellen Cole) Harrington Park Press, an imprint of The Haworth Press, Inc., 1995, pp. 33-44. Multiple copies of this article/chapter may be purchased from The Haworth Document Delivery Center [1-800-3-HAWORTH; 9:00 a.m. - 5:00 p.m. (EST)].

stand patriarchy and other systems of domination as sin, creating alienation and oppression in different ways for women and for men.

Classical Christianity has seen 'sin' as a condition of alienation from God, rooted in a primordial 'fall,' which we inherit biologically. The possibility of being rescued from this alienation from God has been laid through the sacrifice of Christ, but we have to include ourselves or be included in that saving event through baptism and personal experience of conversion. We can then grow in grace through being incorporated into this new life in Christ. This is the traditional Christian prescription for 'soul-making.'

My view of sin and conversion differs from this classical view. I view human capacities as ambivalent rather than depraved or in an irreparable condition of alienation. I prefer the traditional Jewish concept of the "two tendencies," the tendency to good and the tendency to evil, and believe that we retain the capacity to choose between them. I also see the good tendency as that which connects us to our authentic existence, our true 'nature,' our 'imago dei.' But I also agree with the view, found somewhat in Judaism, but developed in Christianity, that our tendency to evil has been biased by historical systems of evil.

The world into which we are born is not neutral, but has been deeply distorted on the side of alienation and violence. We are socialized from infancy to conform to those systems, as if they were normal, natural and the will of God. Thus in order to find the right path to spiritual health, we not only have to confront our own sadistic and masochistic tendencies, but also have to unmask the claims of the dominant culture that misleads us about the nature of good and evil. This can mean struggling against persons and institutions, such as family, school, church, and country, that are close to us, that call for our allegiance and will be somewhere between disappointed and hostile to us if we choose a dissenting path.

My understanding of what sin is does not begin with the concept of alienation from God, a concept which strikes me as either meaningless or highly misleading to most people today. I think we need to start with alienation from one another. We can then go on to understand how alienation from one another expresses itself in personal relations and social relations of negation of others, as well as self-negation, that are sick-making and violent.

We can then look at the larger systems of social power and culture that reenforce these patterns. Today we have to understand such patterns of destructivity, not only in terms of society, but also in relation to the sustaining environment of nature. Patterns of injustice not only destroy society, they also devastate the earth. It is in this expanded understanding of alienation that we might begin to grasp anew what alienation from God might mean; that is to say, alienation from the very source and sustaining matrix of life itself.

Christians have for too long mixed up the concept of evil as sin with problems of finitude and mortality. Natural limitations should be seen as sources of tragedy, but not the result of sin. What is appropriately called sin belongs to that sphere of human freedom where we have the possibility of enhancing life or stifling it. When this freedom is misused, patterns and organizational systems of relationship are generated where competitive hatred builds up. This violence is sustained both by the egoistic refusal of mutuality, but also by passive acquiesence to victimization of others or of ourselves.

The central issue of sin as distinct from finitude, as I see it, is the misuse of freedom to exploit humans and other earth-creatures and thus to violate the basic relations that sustain life; physically, psychically and spiritually. Life is sustained by a biotic relationality in which the whole attains well-being through mutually affirming interdependency. This is a fancy way of saying that life is sustained by love. When one part of any relationship exalts itself at the expense of other parts, life is diminished for these others. Ultimately the exploiters also diminish the quality of their own life as well, although material profit may abound for them. An expanding cycle of violence is generated.

Sin as distorted relationship has three dimensions: there is a personal-interpersonal dimension, a social-historical dimension and an ideological-cultural dimension. It is imperative to give due recognition to all three dimensions, and not only to focus on the personal-interpersonal aspect, as our confessional and therapeutic traditions have generally done.

On the interpersonal level, sin is the distortion of relationship by which some persons absolutize their rights to life and potency at the expense of others with whom they are interdependent. Thus, for example, in male-female relations men were exalted as those persons in the family system with the superior right to be valued, to receive education in preparation for gainful economic roles and political participation in society. Women were accordingly disvalued. They were denied these advantages of self-development in order to function as auxiliaries to male development.

Christianity was not entirely wrong in seeing the heart of sin as pride, an egoistic selfishness that reduces all others to objectified instrumentality. But it has defined this wrong relationship primarily *vis à vis* God, and thus failed to develop the implications of this teaching for relations to other people. Although pride is certainly an element in distorted relationship, I suggest that this is an unhelpful beginning point, particularly for women and for those men who have primarily been on the underside of systems of privilege. But even for those men who appear fairly advantaged, issues of insecurity and fear of vulnerability need to be recognized.

What is called pride, not to be confused with healthy self-esteem, is generally a cover-up for deep-seated dis-ease with oneself. Moreover, the prideful claims of superiority and privilege of some persons and groups over others can only be maintained by some combination of coercive repression and cooptation of these others. In one way or another one must force the victims to acquiesce to and even become collaborators in their own victimization. Aggressive pride can abound only when fed by passive acquiescence of most others, and the ability to isolate enemies who can be violently coerced into subjugation. One has to see all these elements of the pathological relationship.

Some of the earlier ventures of feminist ethics suggested that women's sins are primarily the sins of passivity, of failure to develop an autonomous self, leaving in place the assumption that men sin primarily through pride. Naming passivity as well as pride as components of sin was a significant advance in ethical understanding of the pathological distortion of relationship, but dividing it neatly by gender is too simple.

Although women have been directed to accept passivity, acquiescence and auxiliary existence to men as 'feminine virtue,' they also exist within class and race hierarchies where they can exercise exploitative hauteur toward those under their power. Women, as well as men in 'advisory' relations, also learn to cultivate passive aggressive or manipulative use of power to control those whom they cannot dominate directly.

Patriarchal masculinity has directed men to develop a self-confident, in-charge relationship to women and others under their power, but such confidence does not come easily. The appearance of confident control covers over insecurity. The deeper this insecurity the more it generates a cycle of violence. The male growing to manhood in patriarchal society was parented as a child largely by women. His masculinity is rooted in the over-throw of the mother who was once the all-powerful presence in his early life.

Thus, I suggest, underneath every assertion of male hegemony over women is the fear of women as the 'great mother.' The more insecure his 'manhood,' the more aggressively he needs to put down his wife in order to secure his emancipation from his mother. The need for totally secure, dominating power characteristic of egoistic aggression feeds on an unsatiated void of an insecure, ungrounded self, with its unresolved fears of vulnerability and dependency.

Although the root of domination in the insecure self is most obvious in gender relations, it lies at the heart of every dominating and exploitative relationship. White racists need continually to repress blacks and punish them for the first signs of 'uppitiness.' Anti-semitic Christians needed to repress and punish Jews in order to secure their claims to be God's new 'chosen people.' Right-wing Israeli Jews need continually to silence Palestinians and to punish their smallest self-expression in order to maintain the claims that the land of Palestine is theirs and theirs exclusively. The militarist needs enemies who justify his demands for ever larger and more total systems of military might.

This cycle of violence is fed by the belief that, if more and more power is gained over the subjugated other, the possibility that they might threaten one's own power will finally be crushed. The other as other will be eliminated altogether, or reshaped as a totally docile instrument of benefit to oneself. But this can never be accomplished, both because the dominating relationship eventually prompts rebellion from the dominated, but also because the dominator himself can only be a dominator through the existence of enemies to be vanquished. This became evident with the recent end of the cold war, where we saw the scramble of the U.S. government military-industrial complex to identify new enemies to justify their arsenals.

But the patterns of domination are not created *de novo* in the movement of privileged males from the nursery to the playing fields to the killing fields. Rather these familial patterns are themselves kept in place and reenforced by the larger historical, social structures in which the family is embedded as a dependent part. We are born into this system of patriarchal relations. We are socialized to accept our roles within it, as males or females, as members of more or less privileged class and racial groups, as if it were normal, natural and the will of God.

This is the inherited, collective, historical dimension of sin, which Christianity called 'original sin,' mistakenly seeing its inheritability as the fruit of sexual reproduction, rather than the historical reproduction of social relations. This is also where sin is experienced as unfreedom, as a power that defines and controls us and which we feel powerless to change, even when we become aware of it as wrong.

We are born into sexist, racist, classist, militarist systems of society. This has shaped who we are from birth, and even before birth, for privilege and unprivilege mean that children may be well or badly nurtured even in the womb due to the availability or lack thereof of good food and medical care for their mothers. Distorted, exploitative relationships are embedded in legal, economic and political systems that define the world around us. This is what the Biblical tradition calls 'the powers and principalities.'

Exploitative social systems are also maintained and reproduced through ideologies which make themselves the hegemonic culture. It is the purpose of this hegemonic culture to make such unjust relationships appear good, natural, inevitable, and even divinely mandated. To question or rebel against such relationships is to rebel against nature and nature's God. Family, school, church, media are all enlisted to socialize both the privileged and the disprivileged to accept their place and role in this system of evil, to interiorize its mandates as their identity and duty.

Yet we are not left without a trace of our 'imago dei,' of our capacity for healthy and life-giving relationality, intimations of which persist in our intuitive sensibilities despite this ideological and social misshaping. Nor are we left without exemplars of good and life-giving relationships in family, friends, mentors in education, religion, work and even sometimes in politics. We inherit critical counter-cultures and communities, the fruit of past transforming movements in society, that hold forth alternative visions.

Culture and society, then, also express the struggle between the 'two tendencies,' the tendency to just and loving relations and the tendency to hostile negation and exploitation of others and of ourselves. How then do we understand growth in the 'good tendency,' or 'soul-making'? We might describe this as the process of enhancing our capacities, both personally and socially, for sustaining just and loving relationality, of curbing and curing fear of and contempt for others and for ourselves.

Soul-making does not lie in splitting our minds from our bodies, our reason from our passions, as though our good tendency lay in our rationality and our bad tendency in our bodies and passions. Nor can we just turn the dualism upside down, trusting impulse and rejecting thought. We need to look at this process wholistically. Soul-making happens through transformative metanoia, which is both sudden insight and also slow maturation of a grounded self in relationship or community, able to be both self-affirming and other-affirming in life-enhancing mutuality. It is both a gift and a task, grace and work.

Such transformative metanoia is both personal and social. It cannot be fulfilled simply as an individual journey, although some individuals seem to accomplish a remarkable depth of soul; of inward tranquility and kindness to others in the midst of hostile relationships. As sin is not a 'something,' a bad 'part of ourselves,' but distorted relationship, so metanoia or soul-making is essentially a journey of transformed relationship, relationship to oneself, to one's immediate community, of society and of culture, finally, a transformation of our relationship to all creation, to animals and plants, air, soil and water. Reconciliation with God is within this whole process of transformation and reconciliation with others. It is what the Biblical tradition calls the 'reign of God.'

Our journeys of metanoia and soul-making will differ both because of the differences of individual histories and because of differences of social context, as males or females, as white, Black, Asian, or other ethnic cultures, as more or less privileged economically. Women within the same general class and culture differ in the extent to which they have been socialized to accept patriarchal mores and abused by its violence. Similarly, patriarchal self-identity has 'taken' with some men more deeply than with others. Family patterns, social environment, as well as differences in 'temperament' that cannot easily be explained by socialization, all play a role in these differences.

To the extent to which these patriarchal patterns have been held lightly, with positive role models of mutuality available, the journey may seem easy or obvious, while the abused woman who has internalized patriarchal sanctions may experience its discrediting as deeply traumatic. She may be precipitated out of its securities only through profound outer crisis in which remaking her inner world becomes necessary for her own personal survival. Some kind of alternative community that provides an alternative culture and world view also is essential for her to embark on this journey.

A woman who experiences dissenting thoughts alone, without any network of communication to support her, can hardly bring such dissent to consciousness. She is cowed into submission by the authorities of family, school, church, etc., that surround her and judge that such dissent is the sign of either sin or craziness or both. Thus only when there is a feminist movement that has been able to establish some foothold, creating an alternative vision of being a woman, developing networks of communication and community, can critical and transformative feminist self-perception come to consciousness and be acted upon in a woman's life. The consciousness-raising groups of 1960s feminism were examples of such communities.

Openness to feminist consciousness demands that the ideology and socialization into 'feminine virtue' be thrown into question. All the ways that women have been taught to be 'pleasing' and 'acceptable' to men are critically reviewed as possible tools of false consciousness and seduction, preventing women from asking who they are as persons. Although feminist parents may try to raise daughters and sons to be egalitarian, it is not easy for individual families to compete with the larger culture. Teen-age and young adult years are a time of strong needs to conform to the peer group and its social references. Thus the deeper journey out of patriarchal consciousness often is one that belongs more to the mature stage of life.

Yet if women comply with traditional female roles well into their adult years, and receive some status and secondary power through this compliance, it also becomes difficult to make this journey. Such women have lost a large part of their lives. They have missed the educational opportunities to develop skills for a more self-defined life. It is painful to face up to their own self-betrayal, as well as betrayal by those with whom they have identified themselves. Such women become ready candidates for anti-feminist crusades.

For Christian women from conservative traditions one of the most difficult barriers to feminist consciousness is the Christian identification of sin with pride and anger and virtue with humility and self-abnegation. They have been told they must always put others, their parents, husband, children, first. For women this view of sin and virtue functions as a powerful reenforcement of female subjugation and lack of self-esteem. Such women feel that rebellious thoughts and self-affirmation are the roots of that sin of Eve for which they must atone by redoubled self-negation, even accepting abuse as the means of salvation. Women are to become 'Christlike' by having no self of their own. They will save themselves and their abusers by accepting exploitation and becoming 'suffering servants.'

In the context of such socialization, the claiming of one's own quest for selfhood seems forbidden territory. Yet the conditions that precipitate such a choice for one's own personhood may be experienced, not only as traumatic, but also as exhilarating. In the classical Christian sense of conversion as an experience of transforming grace from beyond our present reality, conversion from sexism is like a gift of power and expanded possibilities.

Part of this breakthrough experience also involves getting in touch with one's own anger and hurt, bringing to consciousness one's experiences of betrayal and abuse and recognizing one's own complicity with this diminishment. This anger also has an energizing element, like a new inner power that allows one to break the chains that have bound you to the culture and systems of sexism.

Consciousness of this personal history also leads to recognition of the collective history of patriarchy and its stategems of enforcing female subjugation. One begins to read, and perhaps write, this collective history in all of its ramifications. One's anger deepens as the fuller collective history comes into view. One should not short-circuit this work of anger, but also one must recognize its dangers, the danger of being stuck in soul-destroying resentment. Thus the unleashing of consciousness of all that has been lost and destroyed needs to become deeply rooted in love, self-love and compassion for others. One needs to move through anger to a deep enough self-esteem to forgive oneself and one's victimizers. To forgive, however, is not to forget, or to capitulate once again into victimization. It is only from a context of a certain confident autonomy, one that also allows some critical distance on one's own capacities to oppress others, that one can rebuild relations with others and with oneself, moving into increased capacity for mutuality.

Such a journey cannot remain only on the personal/interpersonal level nor can it develop simply as consciousness without praxis. It needs to be actualized in action. A woman may decide to seek additional education in preparation for new arenas of life. In so doing relations with significant others will be transformed, or perhaps broken. In the process new awareness of the workings of the structures and ideology of patriarchy comes to be recognized.

But the journey of feminist soul-making must also break out beyond the boundaries of the personal journey and become a journey in solidarity with others, others of one's own group and also others across class and race. This recognition that one's own liberation is an integral part of the liberation of a community, a people, comes much more readily to women of oppressed races and groups. The ideological and cultural encapsulation of middle class white people, women as well as men, make it much more difficult to see beyond the personal/inter-personal arena.

Yet, as women seeking liberation enter into this larger struggle for liberation, they also recognize more fully who they are. When a woman is a person of some class and race privilege, she must also take account of her own capacity to victimize others or simply to be the unconscious recipient of benefits based on their exploitation. One becomes more aware of the ways that the victim too learns to victimize others. This critical distance on one's own context, however, must also become a committed and compassionate praxis, a praxis of solidarity that seeks to ameliorate the systems of exploitation that perpetuate the cycle of violence.

Parallel to the female journey into liberation from patriarchy there also needs to be a male journey. I do not attempt to chart its process here. The fuller description of its dynamics awaits a mature men's movement. Much of what is passing for 'the men's movement' at the moment does not yet seem to me to qualify for such a mature movement of men against patriarchy, but has many features of reduplication of male patriarchal identities and relationships.

A mature men's movement can only arise among men who have been willing to listen to women's story long enough to care deeply about what has happened to women under patriarchy, to have become compassionate enough to support women's journey into an autonomy that can allow genuine peer relations between men and women, and also courageous enough to risk ridicule and censure from other men when one breaks with patriarchal sanctions. A mature men's movement would also recognize that it has to move beyond the personal/inter-personal context toward a struggle for transformation of the larger social structures of injustice.

The journey of 'soul-making' is incomplete without a transformation of the whole. To adapt Augustine's language, our hearts are restless until we rest in this whole. Unlike Augustine, however, we cannot split reconciliation with God from reconciliation with all the others with whom we are interdependent. Indeed our hearts must remain restless, and stir up restlessness anew, as long as women are raped, children beaten, men sent to war, animals are tortured to make them our meat. To remain in compassionate relation to all others who suffer is not simply a gracious choice of the saint, but a necessity of our reality. To 'bliss-out' by oneself in the midst of a suffering world is denial of one's own reality, one's interdependency and complicity with this suffering.

Yet, since total transformation and reconciliation will never be fully accomplished within history, since the reign of God is an eschatological norm, not a historical possibility, since both tragedy and sin will continue, hopefully partially alleviated by our struggles for personal and social metanoia, we also have to learn to sustain our soul-making in our personal and social relationships in the midst of defeat. We have to taste wholeness in the midst of the insufficiencies and tragedies of natural life, of the child born brain-damaged, the young man inexplicably stricken down by disease in the prime of life. We also have to sustain our faith, hope and capacity for love in the midst of cruel reversals of our best efforts, victories betrayed and the martyrdom of prophets.

Soul-making takes place in and through the cross, yet in spite of the cross. The cross is not our goal. Christians must cure themselves of a masochistic spirituality that glories in suffering, usually prescribing it as a way of perfection to be endured by those already victimized. Natural suffering, or tragedy, and unnatural suffering, or unjust violence, are neither the goal nor the way of soul-making, but they are the context in which we must endure and keep the faith in healing love, despite the presence of its contradictions.

The journey of soul-making in community is a never completed or perfected process. There will be no millennium where it is established 'once-for-all' in static perfection. Rather we must take up the task in each day, in each relationship, in each generation, in specific social and historical contexts; the struggle to enhance loving, truthful and just relationships and to curb and cure hate, fear and violence. It is in this way that we also both receive and manifest the redemptive work of the Holy One.

Letter to a Friend:
A Reflection on Connectedness
and Naming

Elizabeth Brosnahan-Broome

SUMMARY. In a letter to her younger friend, Elizabeth reflects on topics that arose when she and Barbara met for lunch. These include the emergent groups of women who gather intentionally to explore their own spirituality, and groups of women who gather and unintentionally create community. She sees the shared power in these groups as being politically opposed to the vested power of the therapist in the psychotherapy dyad. Models of "mentally healthy" females are to be found in the writings of feminists whose works emerge from the socio-cultural and economic matrix of their own experiences.

Elizabeth Brosnahan-Broome, PhD, is a clinical psychologist and educator whose current research projects include the effect of the research on the researcher and phenomenological reflection as a hermeneutic method.

Address correspondence to the author at 3947 Clayton Avenue, Los Angeles, CA 90027.

[Haworth co-indexing entry note]: "Letter to a Friend: A Reflection on Connectedness and Naming." Brosnahan-Broome, Elizabeth. Co-published simultaneously in *Women & Therapy* (The Haworth Press, Inc.) Vol. 16, No. 2/3, 1995, pp. 45-53; and: *Women's Spirituality, Women's Lives* (ed: Judith Ochshorn, and Ellen Cole) The Haworth Press, Inc., 1995, pp. 45-53; and: *Women's Spirituality, Women's Lives* (ed: Judith Ochshorn, and Ellen Cole) Harrington Park Press, an imprint of The Haworth Press, Inc., 1995, pp. 45-53. Multiple copies of this article/chapter may be purchased from The Haworth Document Delivery Center [1-800-3-HAWORTH; 9:00 a.m. - 5:00 p.m. (EST)].

Thursday 8 p.m.

Dear Barbara,

I have been thinking a lot about our conversation at lunch two weeks ago. I am always surprised at how easily we come together after months of not seeing each other. Of course, our sporadic correspondence in-between-times helps.

I can't believe you are going to start your third year of law school. (Is that the sort of thing your *mother* would say?) By the time you graduate, I just might get the definition of "tort" into my head. You are awfully patient to tell and tell again what that is.

Remember when we were talking about the lecture on Jung and archetypes that I am to give to that class in the feminist spirituality program and both of us ended up puzzled by the term "feminist spirituality"? I think I come the closest to whatever I mean by that when I am in a conversation with women I like. (I also may love them; but, the adumbrations that appear when I say to someone "I *like* you" are more meaningful to me right now than to say "I love you." "Love" can have such overarching, semi-transcendent connotations. "Like," on the other hand, is concrete. I "like" the way you chop onions. I "like" the way you organize your desk and I "like" your energy.)

Talking with women. *Yes.* Barbara Friedman (1993) wrote: "The essence of female spirituality is wholeness, inclusiveness. It is not about a spirituality for women. It is about Eros; love and connection. . . . The female knows, not with the head alone, but with the whole self" (p.11). At age 60, I can vouch for this.

"Spirituality," the way I mean it, belongs in the realm of the affective domain–much like what Heidegger termed "mood." He said we always find ourselves in the world in one or another mood; that to-be-in-the-world "is never colorless; it is deeply penetrated by a color of one or another ontological mood; we always *are* in a mood-like way" (cited in Vycinas, 1961, p. 43).

This coloration or affective attitude influences everything we do in life. It is the condition of the existential, reflecting ego. Thus, every human task is colored by mood which "orients perception and action at the same time; it operates as an agent of thematization of perception, of selection of information, and of organization of behavior" (Mucchielli, 1972, p. 33).

I'll be interested to know if you think this is an operational description of how one's spirituality "works"; I think its content is beside the point.

Time to move the sprinkler from the lemon tree to my poor sickly geraniums. Do you think it will ever rain again? More later.

Saturday 9:14 a.m. I have been talking with friends about the women's groups that seem to have been formalized over the last four or five years and for a lot of my friends these groups have taken the place of their going to a psychotherapist. Women have become and continue to become more and more political and because of this I believe that the one-to-one very private relationship of a woman with her therapist doesn't work any more for a lot of us. In addition, we are a lot less interested in a relationship where one person, the therapist, holds all the power.

And you said you have joined a group of women who meet with women professors at your law school. Now, I know that your agenda is different from the ones in many of the groups, but, isn't the whole point to be *connected* with others (with the subtexts of: pleasure, increased self-knowledge, decreased feeling of alienation)? To create—when we know we will be in a place for an extended length of time—a sense of community? I read some place that there are "intentional" (self-explanatory) and "unintentional" communities.

It's the "unintentional" ones that fascinate me. Furman (1993), a social ethicist in Chicago, wrote a dynamite paper exploring the unintentional community among older Jewish women at a neighborhood beauty shop. She teased out the following as "mechanisms and styles of social support":–Illness-talk–Discursive Detail (in conversation the women go into great detail [which sends a 'metamessage of rapport and caring'])–Concern and Affection–Humor–Food–Jewishness. She concludes " . . . this unintentional community of women variously provides social support and consequently feelings of social connectedness and self-worth to the participants" (p. 12).

I can take my experiences, slightly modify the language of Furman's categories, and agree wholeheartedly with her conclusions.

Looking at these groups, it makes sense that women are finding participation in them "therapeutic." There is trust, connectedness, acquisition of self-knowledge, ritual–all are components of psychotherapy. But the important thing I see is that unlike the relationship between therapist and client–where the power resides in the therapist–these women share the power in these groups. Another plus in the Jewish group: the price of having a manicure or a hair-do once a week certainly is cheaper than the price of a therapy session in the L.A. market.

Sunday 11:30 a.m. Went to the market this morning–8 a.m.– while most of Hollywood is still in bed. As I was picking up bottled water, D batteries, tins of tuna to replenish my earthquake preparedness backpack that I keep in the trunk of my car, I thought: reminds me of being in a market in Pasadena April 1992, the day of the civil uprising resulting from the Rodney King verdict. I was indeed, that day, picking up water, etc., when I thought: "Geez. I'm doing earthquake stuff. I wonder what I should get for a riot." Then I figured: pick your disaster; the equipment is generic. And with that smartass series of remarks, realized I was very anxious about heading home toward the fires in my neighborhood.

I don't have any African-American women friends. So, when I say: I don't know how they can stand the political, economic, societal crap they get–I really don't know. I was in a feminist theology class with two African-American women; one of them made it quite clear she was sick of being asked by her Anglo classmates that she represent the experiences and point of view of "all black women." In one context though, she did give the example of being with her young daughter and being followed around by the clerk in a small store *because* they were black and thus suspicious persons. She was enraged. Demanded to see the manager. And got denials of course . . . even though a white woman there at the same time wasn't being trailed. And the irony of it all was that the store was one of those non-profits, dedicated to raising funds for the "children of the world."

In the early '60s I was at Fordham in graduate school. I wore the full habit of a nun; coif, veil, inner sleeves. I spent a lot of time in Manhattan going to museums and going to movies. When a woman is dressed in this "unusual" outfit, she certainly is externally visible, but personally invisible. The responses I got from bus drivers, people in restaurants, people on the street, varied from reverence to mumbled curses. And I was struck by the impersonalness of the responses. They had nothing to do with me, Elizabeth. This of course is the experience of receiving what psychologists and everybody else (post-Freudians that we all are) call: projections.

That was the closest I could ever come to the experience of being black in America. And of course, it can be taken as a stupid example, because obviously a white woman could take off the religious habit and blend right in most places. And the privileges that came with the garb more than offset the discomfort of being cursed at for how one looked. I mean, after all, belonging to the American religious class certainly doesn't have much of anything to do with poverty!

So: I buy the books written by women of color and sit reading on my white middle-class porch wondering: how do they stand it. . . .

Just came across a poem of Ruth Forman's (1993). It's so wonderful, here is part of it as a present:

> . . . poetry should ride the bus
> in a fat woman's Safeway bag
> between the greens n chicken wings
> to be served with Tuesday's dinner. . . . (p.10)

Is that a great image or what! Poetry in a market bag, as ordinary and as essential as groceries.

Monday After Work. When it comes right down to it: poets are the women who pare away the inessentials. Poets are the women who cut through dogma (remember the button: "My karma ran over your dogma"! Still makes me laugh). Poets are the women who name "it"–whatever the experience is that we need re-framed for us. Give us back to us without the patriarchal flimflam.

The connectedness with the other, with the natural and the creative world, that typifies feminist writings touches me most directly through the poetry of women. Their images make me laugh, gasp, shake my head in awe at how they language experience. To read feminist texts by women of any color, culture, age, class–I feel like I'm home.

Tuesday Night! Hooray! Holiday Tomorrow! O.K.: here's what I think in regard to the issue we raised about our mutual acquaintance who says she is a feminist Jungian therapist. Current psychotherapies using the techniques of diagnosis, treatment plan, interpretation, and symbolic language, which are being employed by psychotherapists today are based on the two depth psychologies: psychoanalytic (Freudian) and analytic (Jungian). Both of these systems (and the psychologies that derive from them) are ultimately reductionistic. That is, because of their theories of the structure of the psyche they see symbols (and symbolic behaviors) as rising from *and* pointing back to certain given instinctual or archetypal sources in the unconscious.

In addition, the matrix of these two depth psychologies is the white, European, male, heterosexual, middle (highly educated) class construction of social reality.

What I find myself having to say in that lecture on Jung/archetype I am preparing is: it is not possible to be a feminist Freudian or a feminist Jungian. (As I wrote that sentence, I was aware of wanting to fudge around with qualifiers like: "for most women . . . ," and "I think . . . " and "probably. . . . " Called wanting to cover my a__. Old undigested qualifiers come out of me like a belch at the oddest times, but *never* when I'm angry.)

Saturday 3 a.m. Got home from a str-r-range dinner party two hours ago, and I'm still wired. So, I thought, since your *30th* birthday is Thursday–and I even have a card for you in which I plan to enclose this massive missive–I'd explore one more topic with you and then get on with the sexy novel I'm writing. (I mean, honey, I have this technicolor movie running through my head. I write it as I go, I direct it, I star in it, I edit it; did I mention that it totally revolves around ME? And that it is *sexy*?)

In light of this, try not to laugh too hard when you read that the final topic I want to explore with you is that old chestnut: THE MENTAL HEALTH OF WOMEN.

As feminists we eschew the dualisms that are taken-for-granted in this society; the *mind body* dichotomy that is a foundational concept in psychiatry is one of the most noxious. Phenomenology offers a way out of this mess because phenomenology does *not* posit that the human being is comprised of two structures: somatic and psychic. Its philosophical anthropology regards the human as a being inextricably co-related with the world, and further, that the human being *is* consciousness by virtue of her/his embodiedness.

This is to say, the human's immediate perception of the world is pre-reflective and pre-cognitive; this foundational level of perception is an imminent form of consciousness. "It is consciousness which is not yet clear, lucid, self-aware and objectifying. Characteristically, it is opaque and ambiguous, and lived bodily rather than known cognitively. Its modus operandi is to grab hold of things around it rather than to objectify and reflect upon them" (Valle & King, 1978, p. 105). It is this pre-reflective relationship with the life-world that is the ground or starting point for all (reflective) knowledge.

And: how do we get to the lived-meaning of this? I am more and more convinced that we look to the novels, poetry, biography, autobiography, essays of women. Because: it is "through *description* [italics added] that the pre-reflective life-world is brought to the level of reflective awareness where it manifests itself as psychological meaning" (Valle & King, 1978, p. 17). The exquisite descriptions of what has been pre-reflective for women are given to us in innumerable works of women, e.g., Sarton's *The Way We Were*, Rich's essays and poetry, Heilbrun's *Writing a Woman's Life, Critical Fictions'* Philomena Mariani, June Jordan's *Civil Wars*.

Anita Hill took what hid in the pre-reflective life-world and brought it to the level of her reflective awareness and thence to the level of reflective awareness of millions of us. When women in the work-place have been told for decades that we were "crazy" to take seriously a little sexual kidding and fondling by men, a lot of us, in our sad desire to belong, opted to not look crazy.

A way out of the old medical paradigm is to stop using its language. I am involved in an experience, more accurately: I am the experience. Then, I find myself thrown into a "moment" of reflection (the beginning of deconstruction) following the experience, then I, in the process of putting it together in a new way (in light of my culture, etc.,) can *name* my own experience rather than be co-opted by Western culture's psychological terminology. Chicana Bernice Zamora (1993) nails it in her poem "So Not to Be Mottled": (Who else but a poet could ever capture in twelve words the female experience in America?!)

You insult me
When you say I'm
Schizophrenic.
My divisions are
Infinite. (p.78)

See, I think the women writers I've named in this letter (and so many I didn't name) have already launched a new model to replace the old medical "mental health" paradigm for women. They demonstrate that when we women stick with and become conscious of the reality of our fundamental *connectedness*–to our embodied consciousness, to others, to food, to water, to animals, to the air, to our sexuality, to our moodedness–that is: and to our experience, and tell it in our own language, we are living out our humanness.

Robin West (1988) says: "Indeed, perhaps the central insight of feminist theory of the last decade has been that women are 'essentially connected,' not 'essentially separate' from the rest of human life, both materially . . . and existentially" (p. 3). But that mainstream jurisprudence is based on a separation thesis, which says that humans are distinct individuals first and then we form relationships and engage in co-operative arrangements with others.

"If," she continues, "by 'human beings' legal theorists mean women as well as men, then the 'separation thesis' is clearly false. If, alternatively, by 'human beings' they mean those for whom the separation thesis is true, then women are not human beings. It's not hard to guess which is meant" (p. 3).

Oy! Makes my socks sag.

Well, dear Barbara: I hope your birthday is graceful. And that you get *many* presents.

Lots of like,
Elizabeth

REFERENCES

Forman, Ruth. (1993.) *We are the young magicians.* Boston: Beacon Press.

Friedman, Barbara. (1993. July-August). Growing female consciousness spurns out-of-control patriarchy. *New directions for women.* p. 11.

Furman, Frida Kerner. (1993). At the beauty shop: unintentional community and 'women's culture' among older Jewish women. Unpublished manuscript.

Mucchielli, Roberto. (1972). *Introduction to structural psychology.* (C.K. Markmann, Trans.) New York: Equinox/Avon.

Valle, Robert & Michael King. (1978). Introduction. *Existential-phenomenological alternatives for psychology.* New York: Oxford University Press.

Vycinas, Vincent. (1961). *Earth and gods.* The Hague: Martinus Nijhoff.

West, Robin. (1988, Winter). Jurisprudence and gender. *University of Chicago law review. 55*(1). pp. 1-72.

Zamora, Bernice. (1993). So not to be mottled. In Tey Diana Rebolledo & Eliana S. Rivero (Eds.), *Infinite divisions: An anthology of Chicana literature.* Tucson: University of Arizona Press.

SECTION II:
THEORETICAL CHALLENGES

There Is a Balm in Gilead:
Black Women and the Black Church
as Agents of a Therapeutic Community

Toinette M. Eugene

SUMMARY. The purpose of this essay is to contribute to the under-standing that mental health problems are often endemic to the life experiences of Black women, and that the ways of womanists within the context of therapeutic Black churches can offer healing responses

Toinette M. Eugene educates future generations for a more peaceful, ecologi-cal society of diverse peoples–racial, cultural, gender, sexual, and differently-abled–for a genuinely pluralistic, cross-cultural existence. She holds a PhD in Religion and Society and is currently Associate Professor of Christian Social Ethics at Garrett-Evangelical Theological Seminary in Evanston, IL.

Address correspondence to the author at Garrett-Evangelical Theological Seminary, 2121 Sheridan Road, Evanston, IL 60201.

[Haworth co-indexing entry note]: "There Is a Balm in Gilead: Black Women and the Black Church as Agents of a Therapeutic Community." Eugene, Toinette M. Co-published simultaneously in *Women & Therapy* (The Haworth Press, Inc.) Vol. 16, No. 2/3, 1995, pp. 55-71; and: *Women's Spirituality, Women's Lives* (ed: Judith Ochshorn, and Ellen Cole) The Haworth Press, Inc., 1995, pp. 55-71; and: *Women's Spirituality, Women's Lives* (ed: Judith Ochshorn, and Ellen Cole) Harrington Park Press, an imprint of The Haworth Press, Inc., 1995, pp. 55-71. Multiple copies of this article/chapter may be purchased from The Haworth Document Delivery Center [1-800-3-HAWORTH; 9:00 a.m. - 5:00 p.m. (EST)].

55

to problems that are occasioned primarily by the oppressive social infrastructures of racism, sexism, and classism. This paper will attempt to draw connections between the political, social, and economic contexts of Black women's lives and "dis-eased" states, and to promote an integrated understanding of the life and mental health experiences of "churched" African American womanists.

INTRODUCTION: REDEFINING WOMANIST RELIGIOUS EXPERIENCE AS A THERAPEUTIC AGENT OF CHANGE

In the preface to her collection of prose entitled *In Search of Our Mothers' Gardens*, Alice Walker (1983) defines a womanist as a Black feminist or feminist of color who, among other things, is willful, serious, loving and "committed to survival and wholeness of entire people, male and female" (p. xi). Walker's use of this folk expression common in African American communities has become the foundational source for identifying womanist theology. This concept has generated attention from theologians and ethicists because it resonates with life and faith experiences of Black women that are clearly in contradistinction to White feminist cultural, social, and theological perspectives (Eugene, 1992a; 1992b).

I argue that the mental health status of African American women is a function of the unique life experiences known by that group as a whole. I hypothesize that the relationship between the quality of life and mental health problems is mediated by psychological distress, anger, depression, and undeveloped political consciousness. My analysis implies that the remedy for these conditions is embedded in the raised consciousness or heightened spirituality of churched African American women and their movement toward social change (Eugene, in press).

Some investigators focusing on issues of race and gender emphasize that social groups must be understood within their own social, economic, and political contexts. For example, scholars have pointed to the need for Black women's own interpretation of their experiences and theories which "explicitly incorporate ethnic and gender identities as a unity" (McComb, 1986, p. 67). McComb's work takes a strong position: alleviating the psychological distress in Black women's lives must involve continuous discovering of who "we" are without the hindrance of mainstream assumptions of "telling them what they are." McComb argues that effectively aiding African American women with psychotherapy means understanding and appreciating the internal psychological constructions of African American womanhood. Research which lacks this perspective is less likely to discover and utilize key interventions, including strong community ties, extended family networks, and reliance on other Black women.

I contend that there are several significant spiritual practices unique to the Black church experience either in form or in content which are undeniably related to the positive mental health status of Black women. These practices can be organized into four possibly therapeutic functions: (1) the articulation of suffering (see Townes, 1993, for a review); (2) the location of persecutors; (3) the provision of asylum for "acting out"; and (4) the validation of life experiences. Also the social organization of the therapeutic Black church and womanist communities of care and support provide for an alternative set of positions which provide self-esteem and role continuity especially for African American women's experience.

Even as I offer the strongest argument that I can for the status of the Black church as a therapeutic asylum and agent for Black women, it is equally important to acknowledge the levels of sexism and patriarchy within this institution which conspire to oppress Black women. These oppressions operate primarily in the name of falsely derived male authoritarian hierarchy determined from faulty scriptural exegesis and from unauthentic theological hermeneutics. James Cone (1984), premier proponent for Black liberation theology, makes this challenge indisputably clear to the credibility of the Black church and this profound flaw in its public praxis in a dictum addressed to Black theology, Black churches, and Black women. In a section of his work entitled "A Word Addressed to Black Male Ministers and Theologians," he emphasizes that:

> It is important for black men to realize that women's liberation is a viable issue. We must recognize it and help others in the church to treat it seriously. It is not a joke. To get others to accept it as an issue that deserves serious consideration and discussion is the first step.
>
> As ministers in the church, how we treat the issue will

affect the attitudes of others in our pastoral care. I realize that many women give the appearance of accepting the place set aside for them by men, as it is still true of many blacks in relation to whites. But just as whites were responsible for creating the social structures that aided black self-hate, so black men are responsible for creating a similar situation among black women in the church . . . It is also important that we learn how to listen to women tell their stories of pain and struggle. The art of listening is not easy, especially for oppressors whose very position of power inhibits them from hearing and understanding anything that contradicts their values. (p. 137)

Cone continues to develop his argument that Black women are in the process of articulating renewed leadership styles and that Black men should support them. He declares that:

It is our responsibility as men to be open to the new styles of ministry that will be quite different from the patriarchal and authoritarian leadership of men. It is our responsibility as men to be open to new styles of ministry and to help our congregations to be open to them. This will involve the necessity of being critical of our brothers who are opposed to women taking leadership positions in church and society. We should be prepared to lose some "friends" as we work for change in the patriarchal structures of black churches and seek to create new ones that are humane and just. (p. 138)

Similarly, preeminent Black church historian C. Eric Lincoln and sociologist of Black religion Lawrence Mamiya posit corresponding views in their epic review, *The Black Church in the African American Experience*:

The prevailing message of black feminism or womanism is that the analytical issues of race and class in the black community can no longer ignore the oppression of sexism. Furthermore, they assert that black clergy and religious leaders should recognize that the existence and survival of black churches is overwhelmingly indebted to the efforts and contributions of women in the pews. If and when these laywomen take up the issue of sexual discrimination in the Black Church, far-reaching changes will occur. (p. 308)

In order to sustain and to make firm the case that African American womanists do experience God within the context of the Black church as profoundly therapeutic as well as liberational, I cite as a paradigmatic case a brief pericope taken from the Pulitzer Prize winning play of Lorraine Hansberry, *A Raisin in the Sun*. At this point in the play the character Beneatha, who is a young adult Black woman, is arguing with her mother about her convictions on the uselessness of God, the church, and religion in general. This powerful emotional scene and confrontation regarding God's existence and influence in this classic work, summarizing the relationship between a mother and daughter, epitomizes the perspective of many womanists' views on God within the context of the Black church as indisputably therapeutic in their own lives.

> Beneatha: Mama, you don't understand. It's all a matter of ideas and God is just one idea I don't accept . . . There is simply no blasted God–there is only man and it is he who makes miracles!
>
> [Mama slaps Beneatha powerfully across her face.]
>
> Mama: Now–you say after me, in my mother's house there is still God. [Pause] In my mother's house there is still God.
>
> Beneatha: In my mother's house there is still God. (Hansberry, 1972, p. 39)

BLACK WOMEN'S THERAPEUTIC AND MENTAL HEALTH CONCERNS

The disadvantages of being Black, poor, and deprived of vital resources not only impair social mobility. They also contribute generously to "excess deaths" among Black Americans. The term refers to the number of deaths in a population that would be expected (the normal amount); in the United States, the "normal" amount is based upon the White population's death rate (Department of Health and Human Services, 1984). Blacks' excess deaths are the number of deaths disproportionately over and above White deaths. Political scholars and commentators have equated these conditions with "genocide"–motivated by political and cultural imperialism favoring White, Western, rational, Protestant patriarchy (Davis, 1990; Marable, 1983). Thus, genocide–the deliberate destruction of a racial, political, or cultural group–is a direct result of Black women's and Black people's status as exploitable internal colonies.

According to Byllye Avery (1990), Director of the Black Women's Health Alliance in Atlanta, Georgia, one manifestation of genocide is violence, the principal health problem of African American women. Violence has multiple meanings and takes various forms. It has shaped the history of African Americans since the institution of slavery began. Violence has robbed the Black woman of her "generations," which she bore only to have them torn from her and sold off into slavery. It necessitated her submission to sexual abuse and beatings at the hands of slave masters. It kept Black families economically unstable and dependent upon the "good will" of a morally bankrupt government and economic system.

Historically and currently violence takes the form of undernutrition, inadequate clothing, homelessness, and overcrowding, and restrictive social welfare policy (Jewell, 1993). Violence also shapes Black women's social relations both inside and outside their own households, involving other family members and acquaintances (White, 1985). This causes feelings of alienation and marginality among Black women, making responses to treatment or therapy more difficult. Additionally, Black women have been victims of violence at the hands of authorities and legal systems which refuse protection to women of color from domestic violence, incest, rape, sexual harassment, gender and race discrimination, lynching, and police brutality (Morton, 1991).

Finally, women's studies literature is replete with examples of women's restricted opportunities to define their own lives, because of fear of victimization. For example, in Alice Walker's Pulitzer

Prize winning novel, *The Color Purple*, the main character, Celie, is threatened with physical abuse by her husband when she attempts to make friends, write or receive letters from her sister, and start her own business.

THERAPEUTIC FUNCTIONS OF WOMANIST COMMUNITIES AND THE BLACK CHURCH

The juncture of womanist communities of care and the therapeutic Black church traditions form a bridge wherein African American women can receive unqualified therapeutic intervention and assistance for which they often stand so much in need as a response to the vicissitudes of life lived in the culture and context of the dominant American culture.

1. Articulation of Suffering: Confronting and Exorcising Evil Through Song

Contemporary African American women use the spirituals (religious songs of the slave ancestors) and gospel music (religious songs of the descendants of the slaves) to praise God, to protest in faith, and to seek civil freedom against structural malevolence. Through the spirituals and gospel music, womanists both express their heritage of communal zeal and demand respect, justice, human freedom, and dignity. Like their predecessors, the 1960s civil rights activists, the 1990s womanists proudly rely on a strong African American heritage reminiscent of the music of the spirituals and of the blues, their secular analogue.

African American spirituals and gospel music are the product of a maieutic or midwifery process (Kirk-Duggan, 1993). These culturally therapeutic artifacts helped incubate and deliver the souls of Black folk from total despair. Spirituals and gospel music disclose the reality of and the fight against two malevolent evils that helped induce their birth: slavery and racism, and their concomitant companions, sexism and classism. If social life is constructed from a collective conversion of gestures and symbols from which shared meanings are derived, creating a situational culture, then the spirituals and gospel music represent a base for communication upon which Black folk have built a collective therapeutic perspective on their situation as oppressed people in America.

Another major function of these songs, a function which has survived into contemporary times as favored by the legendary gospel singer Mahalia Jackson and by the incomparable blues singer Billie Holliday and others, is the legitimate collective expression of the suffering experienced by Black women in America. It is this articulation of suffering through music and speech which seems to have a major therapeutic function within the womanist and larger Black community.

In attempting to reconcile the labeling theory of mental illness with the reality of mental stress and personal and social change, Thomas Scheff (1975), in *Labeling Madness*, links the repression of emotion to the creation of an adult who is well adjusted to the social situation in which hierarchy, order, and predictability are emphasized. For Black culture to produce an adult who is well suited to this type of human situation would be to produce a people unwilling to struggle for change and therefore willing to accept their downtrodden and oppressed lot in American society. In support of his corollary to the labeling theory of mental illness, Scheff describes a "speak bitterness" session in the People's Republic of China:

> People confessed, not their sins, but their sorrows. This had the effect of creating emotional solidarity. For when people poured out their sorrows to each other, they realized they were together on the same sad voyage through life, and from recognition of this they drew closer to one another, achieved common sentiments, took sustenance and hope. (p. 86)

Scheff also mentions that this type of social form can also be found in fundamentalist churches and in Black churches in the United States. Such meetings:

> Stimulate collective catharsis in such a way that the needs of individuals to release tension or distressful emotion are met. At the same time, this collective catharsis gives rise to heightened solidarity and a sense of cultural community within the

group. As long as this form leads to genuine and spontaneous emotional release, it serves a vital need for the members and develops an extremely cohesive group. (p. 86)

In many therapeutic Black churches this type of session occurs in the evening prayer meetings. In this setting, many womanist members of the church recount sources of suffering in their lives and ask for prayers by the membership to alleviate their sufferings. They ask for help in bearing their burdens in the same manner as Jesus did in order not to be crushed by them. Prayers recount collective situations of suffering, many times referring to the tiredness of body that overtakes Black women because of the type of occupations in which they work.

The songs sung are also accounts of suffering which symbolically represent the sufferings of all Black people. James Cone (1972) describes how Jesus and God are not distinct entities within the Black church (see Grant, 1989). It is not that he is just "the deliverer of humanity from unjust suffering" (p. 47) or a "comforter in time of trouble" (p. 47) but also someone to whom Black women can tell all about their troubles because he suffered also. Jesus is pictured as the Oppressed One who could do almost anything. When various members in prayer meetings or revivals pray or testify, the congregation usually shares the account of their suffering with numerous "amens" and "tell Jesus." It is at once a communication to fellow members that they understand their troubles and a way of communication to God that this sister's trouble is like their own.

Choirs and gospel singers also depict the past and present suffering of Blacks in the rural and urban settings. Not only do men and women weep at these concerts, but a good number of them also faint, shout, and cry out "thank you" to Jesus for helping them endure. The singing is a representation of accounts of suffering endured personally and collectively; insults –"everybody talkin' 'bout me"– and scorn are sung about. Besides the endurance of suffering there is an expression of aloneness that Blacks have endured, overcome, and will overcome.

2. Locating the Persecutors

Womanist communities in the therapeutic Black church, particularly, are able to avail themselves of the forum of prayer meeting to talk about their troubles with their husbands, partners, and sons. They ask not only for the collective support of the membership in helping them to endure their personal trouble–an arrest, a lost job, a drinking problem, a drug problem, and even an adulterous affair– but they also ask the prayers of the membership in changing the behavior of the persons responsible for the trouble. It is a very pragmatic form of prayer and testimony. The prayers toward the end of the service can range from pleas for effecting a change in an erring son or husband's behavior to a prayer that the family may be able to endure a struggle against "that racist policeman" or "that racist store owner."

Not only are prayers offered up against the offender, plans of action may be formulated to attempt to change the offending behavior. Ministers or members may pay visits to the offending spouse, bail money may be raised. Peer pressure, therefore, can be an extra benefit. If the problem is no food on the table because of a welfare worker, food may be provided, as well as clothing. There is the notion and belief that suffering accounted for is caused by the acts of real persons in the real world, and the right to "tell God all about our troubles" means just that–all of our troubles.

When problems arise such as unwed motherhood and divorce, the prayer meeting is both a forum for announcing the impending trouble and for gathering the social supports necessary to endure and to actively cope with the situation. Church members may render various forms of social support besides prayer. Church members may organize baby showers for an "errant" daughter, thus removing some of the punitive social pressure from the stricken family. Also ministers in the Black church regularly christen or bless the child born of an unwed mother, including the grandparents in the ritual so that the child is made a member of the community and the grandparents (usually a single grandmother) are socially supported in their new responsibility. Although these practices may not depress the rates of social disorganization, they do have the effect of alleviating the personal disorganization which can attend these occurrences. Black divorce, separation, and illegitimacy rates may be public issues, but they are not necessarily personal troubles to be suffered through and endured alone by womanists.

3. Black Womanists and the Black Church as Therapeutic Agents and Asylums

There are very few appropriate settings in American society where one can go specifically to discuss one's personal troubles. The affluent have access to various kinds of therapy groups. Again, it is the affluent and the medically insured who can avail themselves voluntarily of the services of a psychiatric social worker or a trusted psychiatrist. Private social agencies tend to screen out those personal troubles with which they have the least success. Given the overall economic status of the Black population in the United States, therapy for Black women is an expensive solution to private troubles with a limited availability (hooks, 1993). Where economic factors do not intervene, cultural factors such as language barriers, divergent life experiences, and family background are also countervailing forces limiting access to therapeutic facilities (Boyd-Franklin, 1989; Carrington, 1980; Murray & Murray, 1981; Smith, 1981; Wimberley, 1991).

Within the context of Scheff's (1966) labeling paradigm which was previously mentioned in the section on the therapeutic articulation of suffering, a major factor in the labeling process is society's overall view that having a psychiatric personal trouble is shameful. Besides mental illness, other aspects of personal disorganization such as alcoholism, illegitimacy, criminal involvement, and marital troubles are also considered shameful. Even in middle-class America, seeking help for personal troubles, therefore, holds punitive overtones. William Ryan (1971) has shown how the inability of many Blacks to hide or disguise their personal pathologies in the same manner as Whites has led to the distorted view of the Black population as pathology ridden and therefore somehow inferior. The "blaming the victim" ideologies enumerated by Ryan reflect a Protestant American value system that sees humans as ruggedly individual masters of their fate. This problem of "shame" and "guilt" over personal troubles is just one consequence of growing up in a society built upon the ideologies of social Darwinism. To some extent, it affects everyone, not just minorities.

I maintain that womanists and some Black churches, those often characterized by extreme emotionalism, provide and are agents and asylums of therapeutic assistance, refuge, and shelter in non-punitive settings within which Black women in particular are able to act-out and work through whatever happens to be troubling them on Sunday morning or at a prayer meeting evening. This "change of mind" which occurs in the church setting has several names within the Black community. In one of the communities in which I was raised, it is called "getting happy." Churches characterized by this type of behavior were known to us as "shouting churches," and those not characterized by this behavior were called "dead churches."

For the White or Black person socialized religiously in mainline White, "high church" denominations, entering one of these shouting churches can be a frightening experience. Men and women scream and cry and leap about. Bodies seem to be racked by uncontrollable spasms of both grief and joy. People, both young and old, leap about in the aisles, dance at the altar, and fall out on the floor. Those not engaged in such behavior usually attend to those who are, to guarantee that they do not hurt themselves or others while expressing their feelings. A pair of elderly women can lead a young woman through her first experience of "getting happy" by forming a little circle around her with their arms while lending both physical and emotional support, verbally encouraging her on with phrases like: "Tell Jesus"–"Let it all out, Child!"–"Tell your troubles to God!"–"Shout!"– and other encouragements. Members of the congregation develop predictable patterns of acting out, such that other members move to assist them before they actually begin to shout. When certain church women begin to cry, people can be seen changing their seats so that friends can provide comfort and remove infants from possible harm. Choir members who "fall out" during the performance are supported by other choir members while additional verses are sung until the singer regains consciousness in order that she may properly finish the song with the choir.

In the process of the service, womanists become therapists for their fellow church members in that they attend to their shouting, encourage them in their feelings, and guard and protect them from possible harm. Every person takes responsibility for the person nearest him or her. Ministers take their cues from the congregation, and act and speak in ways which encourage such behavior. Choir directors also gauge the length of a song or the number of songs according to the amount of shouting and clapping that is taking place. It is a collective therapeutic experience. The congregation is actively encouraged to lay its burdens on the altar, and it does.

Participants are guarded, welcomed, and sheltered. A woman's shouting is rarely discussed outside the church, although impersonal gossip or particularly legendary episodes may travel about the community and across generations. Legends abound concerning particular incidents associated with famous gospel singers. However, womanist communities and the religious folklore of the Black church supports the social institution of shouting and defines it as good.

Similarly, R. D. Laing (1967), in discussing his idea of the nonpunitive therapy setting, suggests that:

> Instead of the mental hospital, a sort of reservicing factory for human breakdowns, we need a place where people can find their way further into inner time and space and back again. Instead of the *degradation* ceremonial of psychiatric examination, diagnosis, and prognostication, we need for those who are ready for it . . . an *initiation* ceremonial, through which the person will be guided with full social encouragement and sanction into inner space and time, by people who have been there and back. (p. 128)

In this place of healing, among the pastors and preachers, there should be some who are guides or healers, who can educt the person from this world and induct her to the other, to guide her in it and to lead her back again. The ministers, choir directors, singers, nurses, ushers, and fellow church members who aid the "shouters" in their getting happy become Afrocentric shamans for this experience. Shamanism is a respected therapeutic vocation in African and Afrocentric religious communities. Shamans are understood as wise persons (male and female) with healing abilities, capable of mediating outer and inner worlds of experience, and who are highly revered spiritual leaders with the power and desire to heal the pain of others (Jamal, 1987; Nobel, 1991; Noll, 1991).

4. Validating Black Womanist Therapeutic Experiences

The feelings of suffering and persecution experienced by Black women in America are not successfully experienced or shared by the wider society (Townes, 1993). What Black women in American society experience as normal everyday racism is hardly noticed by Whites, or if noticed, it is denied (see hooks, 1992). Much of White America does not see, feel, or think that a wrong has been done and is still being done. It does not understand that compensation, justice, and change are necessary (see Davis, 1983; 1989). In order to maintain their sense of reality in American society, Black women must continuously disregard the official definitions of public events which affect their lives. Sometimes feelings of self-blame can only be blocked by some sort of public, yet in-group, accounting of troubles. The Black church and womanist communities represent the most stable and resourceful institution for providing this function.

CONCLUSIONS

One of the most crucial facts about Black women in the United States is that they have been subject to traumatic experiences involving abrupt cultural transformations (see Eugene, 1989). These occurrences have had serious implications for the disruption of social institutions of the race and for the ways in which Black women have attempted to meet and adapt to these abrupt changes in their lives. The institutions which Black women have had to rely on in bridging these transitional periods were the church and womanist communities of care. Improvisation was required, and these communities of healing were incomparable improvisers.

To be able to know that her troubles are not the result of personal defects; that her inferiority is not a certifiable fact; and that people in certain positions in White society are actively persecuting her, prevents the disjuncture between personal experience and feelings for Black women, and the realities with which they are coping–which for many other people renders them vulnerable to incarceration within institutions for the insane. Womanist communities of care and the Black church as therapeutic agents validate the experiences and feelings that the media of the wider society attempts to invalidate. Because of their differential social organizations, these therapeutic communities provide a sphere of activities in which Black women can perform, function, feel, and express themselves without the invidious distinctions which White judgments bring to bear.

If positive mental health is defined as command of the environment, self-actualization, self-esteem, integration of the self, autonomy within community, and adequate perception of reality, then womanist communities of care and the therapeutic Black church represent social institutions, agents, and asylums which act as irreplaceable supports to the sanity of Black women. Given the crisis of mental health delivery systems and care in America, and the miracle of Black women's survival in America, sensitive and systematic exploration of the possibly therapeutic functions of the religious experience and spirituality of womanists is strongly warranted.

AUTHOR NOTE

Dr. Eugene is the author of *Lifting as We Climb: A Womanist Ethic of Care* (Nashville: Abingdon Press, 1995), and co-author with James N. Poling, *Balm for Gilead: Pastoral Care for African American Families Experiencing Abuse* (Nashville: Abingdon Press, 1994).

The author expresses appreciation to Judith S. Lichtenstein, MD, and Theresa A. Nollette, LCSW, for their invaluable assistance and support in the development of this article.

REFERENCES

Avery, B. (1990). Breathing life into ourselves: The evolution of the National Black Women's Health Project. In E.C. White (Ed.) *The Black Women's health book: Speaking for ourselves* (pp. 4-10). Seattle: Seal Press.

Boyd-Franklin, N. (1989). *Black families in therapy: A multisystems approach.* NY: Guilford Press.

Carrington, C. (1980). Depression in Black women: A theoretical appraisal. In L.F. Rodgers-Rose (Ed.) *The Black woman* (pp. 265-272). Beverly Hills, CA: Sage Publishing Co.

Cone, J.H. (1972). *The spirituals and the blues.* Minneapolis, MN: Seabury Press.

Cone, J.H. (1984). *For my people: Black theology and the Black church.* Maryknoll: Orbis.

Davis, A. (1983). *Women, race, and class*. NY: Vintage Books.

Davis, A. (1989). *Women, culture, and politics*. NY: Random House.

Davis, A. (1990). Sick and tired and being sick and tired: The politics of Black women's health. In E.C. White (Ed.) *The Black women's health book: Speaking for ourselves* (pp. 18-26). Seattle: Seal Press.

Department of Health and Human Services (1984). *Report of the secretary's task force on Black and minority health*. Volume 1, Executive Summary.

Eugene, T.M. (1989). Sometimes I feel like a motherless child: The call and response for a liberational ethic of care by Black feminists. In M. Brabeck (Eds.) *Who cares: Theory, research, and educational implications of the ethic of care*. NY: Praeger Publishing Co.

Eugene, T.M. (1992a). On difference and the dream of feminist pluralism. *Journal of Feminist Studies in Religion, 8*, 91-98.

Eugene, T.M. (1992b). To be of use: Teaching the womanist idea. *Journal of Feminist Studies in Religion, 8*, 138-147.

Eugene, T.M. (in press). No defect here: A Black Roman Catholic womanist reflection on a spirituality of survival. In A. Lumis, A. Stokes, & M.T. Winter (Eds.) *Defecting in place: Woman's spiritual support groups and their challenge to churches*. NY: Crossroad.

Grant, J. (1989). *White women's Christ and Black women's Jesus: Feminist christology and womanist response*. Atlanta, GA: Scholar's Press.

Hansberry, L. (1972). *A raisin in the sun*. NY: Random House.

hooks, b. (1992). *Black looks: Race and representation*. Boston: South End Press.

hooks, b. (1993). *Sisters of the yam: Black women and self-recovery*. Boston: South End Press.

Jamal, M. (1987). *Shape shifters: Shaman women in contemporary society*. London: Arkana.

Jewell, K.S. (1993). *From mammy to Miss America and beyond: Cultural images and the shaping of U.S. social policy*. NY: Routledge.

Kirk-Duggan, C. (1993). African-American spirituals. In E.M. Townes (Ed.) *A troubling in my soul: Womanist perspectives on evil and suffering*. Maryknoll: Orbis.

Laing, R.D. (1967). *The politics of experience*. NY: Ballentine.

Lincoln, C.E., & Mamiya, L. (1990). *The Black church in the African American experience*. Durham, NC: Duke University Press.

McComb, H.G. (1986). The application of an individual/collective model to the psychology of Black women. *Women & Therapy, 5*, 67-80.

Morton, P. (1991). *Disfigured images: The historical assault on Afro-American women*. NY: Praeger Publishing Co.

Murray, S., & Murray, S.R. (1981) (Eds.) *Psychology of Women Quarterly*, Special Issue on African American women, *6* (3).

Noble, V. (1991). *Shakti women: Feeling our fire, healing our world--The new female shamanism*. San Francisco: Harper San Francisco.

Noll, J.E. (1991). *Company of prophets: African American psychics, healers, and visionaries*. St. Paul, MN: Llewellyn Publications.

Ryan, W. (1971). *Blaming the victim.* NY: Random House.

Scheff, T. (1966). *Being mentally ill: A sociological theory* (pp. 55-101). NY: Aldine.

Scheff, T. (1975). *Labelling madness.* NY: Prentice-Hall.

Smith, E. (1981). Mental health and service delivery systems for Black women. *Journal of Black Studies, 12,* 126-141.

Townes, E.M. (1993) (Ed.) *A troubling in my soul: Womanist perspectives on evil and suffering.* Maryknoll: Orbis.

Walker, A. (1983). *The color purple.* London: The Women's Press.

Walker, A. (1983). *In search of our mother' gardens.* NY: Harcourt, Brace, Jovanovich.

White, E.C. (1985). *Chain, chain, chain: For Black women dealing with physical and emotional abuse.* Seattle: Seal Press.

Wimberley, E.P. (1991). *African American pastoral care.* Nashville, TN: Abingdon Press.

Social and Spiritual Reconstruction of Self Within a Feminist Jewish Community

Barbara E. Breitman

SUMMARY. In recent decades, there has been an enormous burst of spiritual energy and creativity among Jewish women. Women have been gathering in a variety of communal forms, some spontaneously generated circles and other more committed long term groups, to create Jewish-feminist ritual, liturgy and theology. The activism, vision, writings, music, poetry and dance of these woman has begun to transform contemporary Judaism. Based on the author's experience in a group that has been meeting for 12 years called B'not Esh, she reflects on how the self can be sanctified, enlarged and at the same time increasingly differentiated over time, through participation in Jewish feminist ritual and community.

"It is not your obligation to complete the task, but neither are you free to desist from it." Pirke Avot II. 21

"The possibilities that exist between two people, or among a group of people, are a kind of alchemy. They are the most interesting thing in life." Adrienne Rich (1972)

Barbara E. Breitman, MSW, is a part-time professor at the University of Pennsylvania School of Social Work and is in private practice at 3900 City Line Avenue, #118D, Philadelphia, PA 19131. She is Co-chair of ALEPH: Alliance for Jewish Renewal, and has led workshops on Jewish identity and the exploration of our Jewish stories at Elat Chayyim: Woodstock Center for Healing and Renewal.

The author wishes to acknowledge, with love, her sisters in B'not Esh and her hope that they will continue to weave visions together for a long time to come.

[Haworth co-indexing entry note]: "Social and Spiritual Reconstruction of Self Within a Feminist Jewish Community." Breitman, Barbara E. Co-published simultaneously in *Women & Therapy* (The Haworth Press, Inc.) Vol. 16, No. 2/3, 1995, pp. 73-82; and: *Women's Spirituality, Women's Lives* (ed: Judith Ochshorn, and Ellen Cole) The Haworth Press, Inc., 1995, pp. 73-82; and: *Women's Spirituality, Women's Lives* (ed: Judith Ochshorn, and Ellen Cole) Harrington Park Press, an imprint of The Haworth Press, Inc., 1995, pp. 73-82. Multiple copies of this article/chapter may be purchased from The Haworth Document Delivery Center [1-800-3-HAWORTH; 9:00 a.m. - 5:00 p.m. (EST)].

A group of 20 Jewish women who have been meeting annually for 12 years sit in a circle on Shabbat morning. We are at a crossroads as a community: our future together is in question. The women who have planned the morning's *davenning* (communal prayer) have designed a ritual to help in the process of transition. They pass around a basket stuffed with rolls of multi-colored fabric, looking like vibrant flowers, and we are each asked to select one. We unfurl the rolls of fabric to find makeshift scarves or prayer-shawls, with strings of wool tied at each of the four corners. They echo in design, but are not meant to replicate, the tallit or tzit-tzit, sacred Jewish prayer garb traditionally worn by men. We sing and chant songs and poems that loosely follow the movement of a Shabbat service, including blessings for the morning, songs of praise, time for meditation.

Midway through the morning, when the *Torah* (Hebrew Bible scroll) would be read in a traditional Jewish service, leaders of the ritual ask us to wander outdoors into the redolent, rural New York springtime, onto the grounds of the retreat center where we are meeting. We are invited to open ourselves to whatever wisdom, whatever '*torah*' (teaching) we can receive about transitions. The night before, a member of the group read to us from a piece she had written about 'crossroads' inspired by the Biblical story of Ruth and Naomi, mother-in-law and daughter-in-law, who find themselves at a crossroads, about to set out on a treacherous journey together. It is a story associated with the holiday of Shavuot, which occurred during the week just prior to our gathering, celebrating God's giving of the Torah at Mount Sinai. According to Jewish legend, all Jews ever to be born stood at the foot of Mount Sinai together in an eternal moment outside of historical time. Thus located in sacred Jewish time, at the intersection of Shabbat with the annual cycle of holidays, we walk silently outside to encounter the natural world.

I pass one woman standing with her arms open wide, chest extended, in a gesture of embrace over a large expanse of field. I see others walk into the woods. Some sit peacefully under a flowered trellis. I am drawn to a newly flowering rhododendron tree, slowly shedding the brown remnants of previous growth as fresh buds emerge on the branch.

When we gather again in the prayer room, we share the stories of our wanderings. One woman has been gifted with the sight of a doe darting between the trees, and seconds later, a fawn leaping closely behind. Another woman speaks of getting lost in the brightness of a single orange poppy standing among a bed of purple irises. A group of women recount their initial anxiety about not getting any 'teachings,' until they discovered each other on the path and ended up in a group embrace. I share the wisdom of the rhododendron tree, noticing how the old growth to be shed co-exists for a long time on the same branch with new buds in various stages of opening and blossoming. Several women recount standing next to the saplings we had planted during our closing ritual two years ago, noticing how they had grown and changed over the years.

Listening to each other deeply, some sharing insights derived from the natural world, some surprisingly moved by the emotional impact of 'discovering each other on the path while out there wandering,' others reflecting on our growth over time, still others musing about our journeys in light of the relationship between Ruth and Naomi, the group intuitively and emotionally wends its way toward a heartfelt recommitment to one another. The leaders invite us to take our shawls and tie them end to end with the corner strings. Standing together, encircled by one long rag-tag shawl, we realize we have done it. We have traversed a crossroads, begun the process of transitioning to a next stage in our groups' development. The ritual has worked. We conclude by singing "L'chi Lach," a song by Debbie Friedman, whose title and refrain translates into the feminine verb form, the famous Biblical exhortation to Abraham to leave the land of his fathers and 'go forth' on his spiritual quest (Gen. 12:1).

These twenty women are members of a group of Jewish women who have been meeting on Memorial Day weekends since 1981 to "re/vision Judaism using the insights of feminist theology and our experiences as Jewish feminists," as explained in the letter of invitation to the first gathering. The group adopted the name B'not Esh ('daughters of fire') in 1983.[1] For me and, I believe, for others in our group, participation over time, in community, in rituals, in discussion and struggle, in celebration, exploring our relationship to Judaism, to feminism, and to each other has enabled both *a social and a spiritual reconstruction of self*, as we have created ways to contribute to a feminist reconstruction of Judaism which includes and takes seriously women's experiences.[2]

Although one could reflect upon the process and accomplishments of this group from many perspectives (Ackelsberg, 1986; Plaskow, 1990), I have been particularly interested, as a feminist therapist, in how the experience of Jewish feminist ritual has enlarged, communalized and sanctified our experiences of self; and how, combined with explorations of group diversity in such areas as sexuality, class, ethnicity, work, motherhood, relationships, the resulting clarifications about the impact of social context on our lives has contributed to individual women's abilities to differentiate themselves from inherited or fixed meanings and self-definitions, to form increasingly distinctive and unique life paths and identities.

Feminist therapists and research psychologists have already amply documented how the concept of the privatized, separate self on which most of Western psychology has been based, has failed to take into account the experiences of women who often sense 'self' as relational, inter-connected with other contiguous selves, embedded in relation rather than separate from it. What even feminist psychology has rarely questioned, however, is the notion of the healthy self as a 'coherent' self, a self in which opposing tensions and tendencies are resolved, in which identity becomes strong by virtue of becoming unitary. What I now believe is that in a non-traditional culture, during a period of rapid social change, in which not only are women's roles increasingly varied, but in which categories of identity (e.g., gender, race, sexuality) are themselves shifting and changing in cultural meaning, the healthy self may rather be a complex self, conscious of multiple identifications co-existing in tension, capable of tolerating contradiction and even fragmentation, highly unique and idiosyncratic.

Living in a larger social context in which we are marginal as Jews, and in a larger Jewish context in which we are marginal as women, B'not Esh has created a spiritual community which places our uniqueness as women and as Jews at the center. This context has enabled individual members to express and develop parts of ourselves, spiritually, sexually, intellectually, emotionally, that had been silenced or repressed in the larger contexts of our lives. My experiences with B'not Esh have enabled me to experience how, at once, the sense of self can be enlarged and collectivized, and how individual selves can become increasingly unique, distinctive, complex and multiple in identifications.

When we truly 'meet' during rituals, individual boundaries are momentarily surrendered, our senses of self expanded, and the shared experience of intimacy in women's prayer community not only creates an experience of enlarged self and empowerment as women, but seems to enable us to feel, alive amongst us, an immanent Presence greater than we are. We experience the sacred ground of the self alive in our midst. When we return to more individuated, self-contained states of being and encounter each other through passionate dialogue about our differences, individual women develop ever more unique and original voices. The group forms a matrix for spiritual transformation and growth.

By remaining in a form of committed, working community over the years, we have broken down the boundaries of culturally structured privatized selves and have experienced communal self, historical and connected to others in both time and space. By choosing to make Shabbas together, we dwell in a kind of eternal time that has been sacred to our ancestors over centuries. By drawing on a multiplicity of metaphors for God, changing the formula Jews have traditionally used to evoke God in prayer, from the masculine and hierarchical "Blessed are You, Lord our God, King of the Universe . . . " to "Let Us Bless the Source of Life . . . ," we reach out to Jewish women of the future, bequeathing them a name for God in whose Image they might find themselves, an image that structures relationship between human and divine as more active and mutual (Falk, 1989). By involving our bodies in movement, dance, and song, opening to experience the homoerotic bonds forming a matrix of energy to sustain women in community, we can feel a sense of kinship with other women of spirit, embodied, praying, dancing in circles all over the world. By engaging in rituals which call upon us to open to the natural world, we reawaken our connection with the Source of Life in nature.

From the beginning, our process of re/visioning Judaism has included both creation and participation in ritual and liturgy, in combination with group discussion. Our discussions have treated as axiomatic the feminist insight, 'the personal is political,' as we continually challenge one another to see the social in the self, to understand the socio-political context of the formation of ourselves. Grappling with our differences has provided an often dissonant counter-point to the unifying harmonies of felt connection that can occur during rituals. As similar as a group of spiritually committed white Jewish feminists might be, we have encountered meaningful differences amongst us. In our group are women of various ages, thusfar able-bodied, some coupled and some single, lesbians, bisexuals, and heterosexuals, mothers and non-mothers, from various class backgrounds, currently living in a range of economic circumstances, Ashkenazi and Sephardi, born Jews and Jew-by-choice. We have struggled, sometimes contentiously, usually trying to expand the domain of honesty between us, as we probe and bring to expression the meanings of these differences. We have "come to recognize issues of process and intragroup relations as crucial to our spiritual task" (Ackelsberg, 1986).

Over the years, we have explored the sociometry of our group in large and small group sessions. We have looked at how our senses of self have been shaped by Jewish text, liturgy, God-language, ritual and historical experience, as well as by gender experiences in families, and communities. Among other issues, we have explored the impact of class differences, the meanings of work, the significance of being mothers and not being mothers, the effects of anti-semitism, our relationships with Israel, the connections between sexuality and spirituality, and the differences in life experiences among lesbian, bi-sexual and heterosexual women. Recently, we have increased the diversity of our membership in terms of age and ethnicity, including younger women and more women of Sephardi and Mizrachi descent; we have also committed ourselves to a long-term, systematic and conscientious process of exploration of diversity issues, including a more extensive look at race and sexuality. Always, our process involves the telling and re-telling of the stories of our lives from many perspectives and angles of vision.

I think many of us feel, as we approach the Bat Mitzvah year of our group, we literally would not be who we are, were it not for our experiences together. Our senses of self and our identities have, in most cases, been profoundly affected by our experiences in Jewish feminist community. This has been particularly true in the areas of spirituality and sexuality. As we have explored how to create a communal setting which truly affirms Jewish women's embodied and spiritual experiences, as we have reflected in discussion on those times in our lives when we felt most fully alive and in touch with something larger than ourselves, we have recognized the inseparable connections between sexuality and spirituality as twin expressions of life energy, of 'the erotic' as Audre Lorde has reclaimed its meaning for feminists. By creating a Jewish context which celebrates the love between women as sacred, B'not Esh has formed a matrix from which several women in the group were enabled to 'come-out' as lesbians, sometimes as lesbian Rabbis, in other parts of their lives. At the same time, women in the group who do not identify as lesbians, participating in a spiritual community which truly affirms the love and bonds between women, have experienced an enlargement in the sense of self to include lesbian experience. This has meant not only taking it as a sacred commitment to act in the world beyond B'not Esh to make other contexts safe and open places in which the love between women can be celebrated; it has meant experiencing the hurt caused by homophobic oppression, as our hurt, experiencing assaults against women loving women, in any form, as assaults against all of us and against the sacred self in which we all participate.

B'not Esh also continually empowers virtually every woman in the group, whether Rabbi or not, to assume spiritual leadership in the community of her choosing. Most Jewish contexts, even if they recognize or legitimate the authority of women leaders, do not provide a context for women to be fully expressive of their spirituality, for women to explore their spirituality, for the uniqueness of the 'woman's voice' as she addresses God to be a central voice in the community. Within B'not Esh, we experience ourselves in community as participating in a much larger process of the emergence of Jewish womenspirit. The enlargement of self that occurs through that process not only sustains us as individuals, beyond B'not Esh, as we participate in a feminist transformation of Judaism, it enables us to carry with us a new sense of possibility for how to be a human self in community and in relationship with the sacred.

From the beginning, feminist thinkers have understood that "each culture constructs a sense of reality and a corollary model of selfhood that it assumes to be either universal or preferable" (Watkins, 1992, p. 52). In the introduction to a collection of essays gathered from a conference on "Feminism/Theory/Politics" in 1985, Elizabeth Weed stated: "The widespread practice of consciousness-raising groups in the 1960s and early 1970s did much to generate one of feminism's most important recognitions: that one's desire may not be one's own, that what one calls one's self may be constructed elsewhere" (Weed, 1989, p. xv). Bronwyn Davies (1992, p. 69), a Professor of Social, Cultural and Curriculum Studies, articulates well how cultural self-structuring contributes to pain and suffering:

> But women's desires are the result of bodily inscription and of metaphors and story lines that catch them up in ways of being/ desiring from which they have no escape unless they can reinscribe, discover new story lines, invert, invent, and break the bounds of the old structures and old discourses . . . it is not the individual woman who is at fault in mistakenly living out a fantasy instead of a reality or for living it incorrectly. It is the culture that has destructive narratives through which identity and desire are organized.

The community of B'not Esh has enabled many of the women involved to "discover new story lines," find a context for the exploration of identities previously suppressed, as we have simultaneously been transforming many of the old structures and the language of Judaism that previously shaped our realities. I have learned with my sisters of B'not Esh that only a process that enables people to explore how cultural narratives have shaped their lives, that helps to unearth and bring to awareness this cultural self-structuring, can make it possible for people to heal from suffering that is culturally generated and choose how to define unique, complex and multi-faceted self(ves) and identity(ies). By creating a social context in which we could honestly explore and affirm aspects of self that are stigmatized or devalued in the broader culture, individual women have been able to take their lives and their work in new directions outside the group.

In a tradition centered around a sacred text made up largely of stories of our ancestors' encounters with the Holy, we have declared our own lives to be the text. As contemporary Jewish women coming to full voice as women of spirit for the first time in our peoples' history, we are claiming that our lives and experiences are part of the ongoing story of the Jewish peoples' encounter with God and therefore of the textual history of Judaism (Alpert, 1991). *In community, we have enabled each other to become women whose struggle to define selfhood is at once a critique of and a contribution to culture* (Watkins, 1992). We are being transformed by the Presence dwelling amongst us at the foot of the mountain.

NOTES

1. Approximately 40 women have participated during the years. Some women have left the community. Members who have participated over the years *and* are currently active as of this writing include: Martha Ackelsberg, Penina Adelman, Rebecca Alpert, Barbara Breitman, Deborah Brin, Betsy Cohen, Sue Elwell, Marcia Falk, Merle Feld, Mary Gendler, Julie Greenberg, Susan Harris, Barbara Johnson, Denni Liebowitz, Jane Litman, Judith Plaskow, Geela Rayzel Raphael, Ilana Schatz, Drorah Setel, Ruth Sohn, Marcia Spiegel, Susan Talve, Esther Ticktin, Ellen Umansky, Shiela Weinberg, Leora Zeitlin, Shoshanna Zonderman.

2. Members have a variety of professional identifications, Rabbi, theologian, professor, therapist, communal service worker, activist, editor, poet, songwriter, educator, health administrator. Among our contributions have been being Rabbis or lay leaders in a range of Jewish communities; founding new feminist and/or Jewish Renewal organizations. Some have written books and articles about Jewish feminism, theology, ritual, history, psychology; some have edited books of poetry by Jewish women or edited feminist and/or lesbian anthologies, written new poetry, plays or translations, composed new blessings, created new liturgies, published books of feminist historical research, composed songs, developed new curriculum on womens' and Jewish issues for adults and children. Some have worked as therapists, educators, and activists in feminist, lesbian, Jewish, communal and/or political organizations in Israel and the United States.

REFERENCES

Ackelsberg, Martha (1986). Spirituality, community, politics: B'not Esh and the feminist reconstruction of judaism. *Journal of Feminist Studies of Religion, 2* (2) 107-120.

Alpert, Rebecca (1991/5751). Our lives *are* the text: Exploring jewish women's rituals, *Bridges*, 2(1). 66-80.

Davies, Bronwyn (1992). Women's subjectivity and feminist stories. In C. Ellis & M. Flaherty (Eds.), *Investigating subjectivity,* xv. New York: Sage Publications.

Falk, Marcia. (1989). Notes on composing a blessing. In J. Plaskow & C. Christ (Eds.), *Weaving the visions: New patterns in feminist spirituality,* 128-138, New York: HarperCollins.

Pirke Aboth: Sayings of the fathers, 62. Trans. R. Travers Herford (1962). New York: Schoeken Books.

Plaskow, Judith (1990). *Standing again at sinai: Judaism from a feminist perspective.* New York: Harper & Row, Publishers.

Rich, Adrienne (1979). *On lies, secrets and silence.* New York: W.W. Norton & Company.

Watkins, Mary (1992). From individualism to the interdependent self. *Psychological Perspectives, 27,* 52-69.

Weed, Elizabeth (1959). Introduction: Terms of reference. In E. Weed (Ed.), *Coming to terms,* New York: Routledge.

Identity, Recovery, and Religious Imperialism: Native American Women and the New Age

Cynthia R. Kasee

SUMMARY. Cultural disintegration and the resulting loss of self-esteem have acted as precursors for rampant substance abuse in indigenous American communities. Especially at risk are Native women, who have little recognition in the dominant culture, but whose traditional roles of respect have also dwindled with forced acculturation. Just when a wave of reconversion (going "back to the blanket") is taking hold among Native women substance users/abusers, the even more prevalent commercialization of Indian religion and pseudo-religion are denigrating these recaptured sources of dignity and pride. This "religious imperialism" doesn't just parody true Native faiths; it robs Native women in recovery of the self-esteem building tool which has proven most effective. It also continues the appropriation of indigenous culture which further serves to undermine coming generations of Native American women.

There is a Cheyenne proverb quoted in Mary Crow Dog's *Lakota Woman* (1990) that says:

Cynthia Kasee is Adjunct Faculty Member at the University of South Florida, Eckerd College, and The Union Institute's Distance Learning Program. She holds an AA in English, a BA in Sociology, and both a BA and a PhD in American Indian Studies.

Correspondence may be addressed to her at the Department of Women's Studies/ISS, HMS 413/468, University of South Florida, 4202 E. Fowler Avenue, Tampa, FL 33620.

[Haworth co-indexing entry note]: "Identity, Recovery, and Religious Imperialism: Native American Women and the New Age." Kasee, Cynthia R. Co-published simultaneously in *Women & Therapy* (The Haworth Press, Inc.) Vol. 16, No. 2/3, 1995, pp. 83-93; and: *Women's Spirituality, Women's Lives* (ed: Judith Ochshorn, and Ellen Cole) The Haworth Press, Inc., 1995, pp. 83-93; and: *Women's Spirituality, Women's Lives* (ed: Judith Ochshorn, and Ellen Cole) Harrington Park Press, an imprint of The Haworth Press, Inc., 1995, pp. 83-93. Multiple copies of this article/chapter may be purchased from The Haworth Document Delivery Center [1-800-3-HAWORTH; 9:00 a.m. - 5:00 p.m. (EST)].

83

A nation is not conquered until
the hearts of its women
are on the ground
Then it is done, no matter
how brave its warriors
nor how strong their weapons. (p. 3)

This has very nearly been the case in Indian Country[1] after five centuries of Euro/American influence. Native women, along with Native men, have seen the loss of land, culture, life and faith. Faith . . . belief . . . religion . . . that thing that most Native languages had no pre-Contact word for, because it was so pervasive it could not be separated from the rest of the indigenous codes of "right living." Faith is the integrating element in Native societies, and at least in its various traditional forms it has served to give meaning to land, culture, life. The forced loss of all the traditional components of Indian life (through warfare, acculturation, boarding schools, missionaries, ad nauseam) is a well-known precursor for the development of modern social pathology. I offer, therefore, that this religious loss has been a major motivator for the rampant increase in abuse of substances and of other people in indigenous communities. Further, the availability of traditional religion is a major motivator for recovery for Indian clients, a process so frequent, it is colloquially referred to as "going back to the blanket."

The loss of culture/religion that has precipitated this explosion of problems has been doubly devastating for the Native woman, as she has borne the brunt of changes in gender expectations as well, changes which have done much to subordinate the Native woman. She originally had much more say-so in her community than pleased missionaries, conquistadors and "Friends of the Indian" alike. Her more equitable role was not emulated by her Euroamerican sisters; it was abhorred, as a possible threat to the prevailing order. Quick work was made to supplant equality with a patriarchal model that alienated her from community/marriage/childrearing decisions, made her body a saleable commodity, and taught her to see a "squaw" in the mirror.

From the Alkali Lake (British Columbia) Reserve to the Peaceful Spirit Sweatlodge, from the Sacred Shawl Society's shelter for battered women to the Minneapolis American Indian Center's many programs for recovery and survival, traditional ways are being offered to the Native woman as a lifeline. She need not become a practicing member of her people's ancient faith to benefit from these programs, but she gains self-esteem from seeing how her ancestral women functioned actively in their religions, governments, clan systems, and marriages. Many of the women who complete these programs *do* go "back to the blanket." The same phenomenon is occurring in prisons throughout the country, where Native women and men are learning a new pride in themselves and their people through a return to tradition. This return carries with it an admonition to not again fall prey to the behaviors that wreaked such havoc in the first place. In these respects, the inner strength and pride that indigenous people develop as a result of this religious reconversion is akin to that of members of the African-American community who have embraced the Bilalian faith or the Nation of Islam.

As we've seen, the loss of traditional religion and its accompanying world-view can lead to anomie, social disintegration, and personal pathology. A return to tradition, at least for Native people and particularly for Native women, can restore the balance, giving pride and recovery a concerted chance to take hold. If such returns to tradition are readily available (and in prisons they often are not available at all), in the Indian helping professions community at least, what is the crux of my argument? Simply said, that amalgam of real and imaginary "Indian religions" which fall under the metaphysical rubric of the "New Age." This movement consists of many elements: meditation, yoga, telepathy, "channeling" of the dead, crystal power, and a number of other occult-identified practices, as well as the commercialized versions of indigenous beliefs to which I allude. Let me be clear; not all "New Agers" practice pseudo-Indian faiths. My disagreement is with those who do. By using the term "New Age," I am also not referring to practitioners of pre-Christian faiths. The untold lives lost to the Witch Hunts correlate with the broken, frozen, bullet-riddled bodies on the snowy field at Wounded Knee. The enforced invisibility of beliefs such as Santeria, Odinism, and Druidism correlate with the hidden Nightway Sings, Bole Maru meetings, and Green Corn Bundle viewings. These pagans are our sisters in the fight, people who have also had to give up much to continue their traditions.

So who really are the New Agers I so strenuously decry? Those who cannot be satisfied with their ancestors' pillage of land, lives and cultures, the ones who must now insist upon taking our god/desses as well. Even those who practice a sort of conscious pan-Indian faith, who readily admit they are creating a smorgasbord of real and imagined Indian beliefs, are "on my list," so to speak. It matters little to me whether they are sincere, misguided people or knowledgeable looters, whether they are non-Indians buying religion or Indians selling it, they are all part of the problem. This is *not* a victimless crime! This hurts all indigenous people, it upsets the balance of the Earth (as some people are responsible for some rituals, while others handle other rituals, and the abandoning of one set for the other tips the scales), and it removes the exclusivity from Native beliefs. While the "franchising" of Indian religions would deal a death blow to cultures practiced collectively by Native people, the loss of group identity conveyed by these faiths would devastate those who also rely on them as the Red Road to recovery. If Indian religions can be bought by any dilettante with a credit card, they lose their ability to require commitment, reform, and diminution of ego. In other words, the practicing Indian Traditionalist is the antithesis of the Ramada Inn Sweatlodge Yuppie.

> They came for our land, for what grew or could be grown on it, for the resources in it, and for our clean air and pure water. They stole our free ways and the best of our leaders, killed in battle or assassinated. And now, after all that, they've come for the very last of our spiritual traditions. They want to rewrite and remake these things, to claim them for themselves. The lies and thefts just never will end. (Churchill, 1992, p. 197)

I do not simply vent my frustration over this religious imperialism in order to find an "other" to blame. There is a time-honored tradition called divide-and-conquer which is at work here. My non-Indian compatriots in feminist circles share with me a central similarity. We are the inheritors of a social order based upon an elitist patriarchy which has marginalized women, people of color, poor people, those differently-abled, gay/lesbian/bisexuals, and the veterans of those conflicts we find embarrassing in retrospect. In addition, we are often "set at" one another in order to minimize the power we might muster as an amalgam. So we are told, for instance, that Affirmative Action favors minorities (read: racial/ethnic minorities), deflecting attention from the fact that the power structure's economic policies continue to reduce the employment base, exacerbating the job-hunter's task. Need a good answer? Blame a minority. It's a short step, often taken, for the average American to turn against whatever the most recent request is that a minority group has made.

It is my belief that feminists engaged in religious imperialism towards Native faiths are dupes of this divide-and-conquer strategy. At least that's what I tell myself. It's more workable than believing that every feminist New Ager is an intentional looter, repeating the pillage methods that left her marginalized and stealing the Red Road to recovery from her Native countrywoman. I do not issue a blanket indictment of feminism either; much has been done recently to include the perspectives *and the concerns* of women of color in feminist circles. Nor do I think there is some Grand Strategy Room where secret committees, their brains awash in testosterone, meet to hatch the latest conspiracy. However, I do cite as evidence the fine, old imperialist policy of maintaining surface friendship with two peoples, while silently aiding them in the annihilation of each other, to the benefit of the powerbroker (Collections, 1897).

If Indian faith continues to be so sadly parodied by "plastic medicine wo/men," it loses its dignity in the eyes of the rest of the world. It is very difficult these days to convince the average American that Native people do not have a constitutional guarantee of religious freedom. Firstly, they do not realize that anyone is excluded under the Constitution. Secondly, they know a place locally where you can go to a retreat house for a weekend and they'll set you up on a vision quest, for a modest sum, of course. "How can *you people* say your religions are endangered when there are plenty of listings in the Yellow Pages for shamans?" (You can hear the patronizing tone in that delivery, can't you?)

The parodying of Native religion diminishes it, creates a plethora of misinformation, and takes the heat off legislators considering yet again whether to grant Indians constitutional guarantee of free practice. In terms of personal loss, the move away from exclusivity in Native practices cuts the legs off the "back to the blanket" movement in Indian recovery. That a person who espouses feminism could do this to another marginalized person, and particularly one in such precarious physical and psychological circumstances, is a cruel betrayal. Consider this, though: cultural genocide, religious imperialism, objectification by gender, divide-and-conquer . . . they all go hand-in-hand, and far too often these days, that hand belongs to someone who calls herself my "sister." She is not. She is aping the behavior taught to her. She is engaging in an extension of the marginalization and oppression which has been done to her by patriarchy. Again, I do not generalize to the entire feminist community; indeed, there are many sisters (and some brothers) in the circle who recognize this hypocrisy.

> It is important to respect the fact that some ceremonial knowledge is sacred and private, meant only for the medicine societies that are responsible for these ceremonies. It is a great offence to exploit sacred knowledge. Proper performance and participation is the duty of designated traditional religious leaders. Many of these ceremonies are site-specific in their respective nations. . . . (Magnuson, 1989, p. 1086)

Am I putting too much emphasis on a recovery tool which is by no means universal or reducible to empiric quantifying? Is the role played by indigenous religions not simply analogy to the Higher Power principle in Twelve Step programs? Can't it then be interchanged with any other quasi-religious principles which require commitment and work with equal efficacy? I would argue that it can't. At least not in the life of the recovering Native woman. Her self-esteem has been decimated by the system put in place by those self-same religious principles touted in Twelve Step programs. The healing power of a return to tradition lies in it being the center of a matrix of group identity elements, all of which must remain indigenous-identified in order to restore to her something her ancestors had. The imperialist "faith grab" is the first step to final cultural genocide.

Within the context of advanced settler-state colonization, however, things have become rather more complex and confusing. Here, members of the dominant culture are unable to retain their sense of distance and separation from that which they dominate. Instead, over a period of generations, they increasingly develop direct ties to the "new land" and, consequently, exhibit an ever-increasing tendency to proclaim themselves "natives." This, of course, equates to a quite literal negation of the very essence and existence of those who are truly indigenous to the colonized locales. (Churchill, 1992, p. 142)

The deepest avatar of racism is to think that an error about (other) societies is politically less serious than a misinterpretation of our own world. Just as a people who oppresses another cannot be free, so a culture that is mistaken about another must be mistaken about itself. (Baudrillard, 1975, pp. 32-3)

That any feminist colludes with the "faith grab" is a devil's bargain with the very forces which have deprived her of so much. That she is willing to do so against a sister doubly oppressed (gender and race) stings much worse than the actions of our common oppressor. That she is willing to do so, knowing that she moves health out of her indigenous sister's reach, negates any other good she may have done on behalf of our gender, or any other group characteristic we may share.

What should you avoid if you are a concerned feminist who has simply not thought of these implications before? Ask what elements of the New Age pseudo-Indian hodgepodge ring false with the most cursory of examinations. Are they charging me for this knowledge? If the answer is "yes," walk the other way. Given the hypothetical situation, if you were, say, a Presbyterian and you wished to take instruction to convert to, say, the Episcopal faith, would you do it at some temporary site, replete with facilities to serve large numbers (thereby reducing overhead and maximizing profit), and only after the payment of a fee? I'm not talking here about retreats, which are common in Christianity; rather, I mean paying for a ceremony which conveys a specific blessing or power. How much does Confirmation cost? How about Baptism/Christening? Granted, a donation may be strongly encouraged, but sincere clergy will not deny you these ceremonies for want of money.

Are they telling me to avoid "real" Indians (i.e., Traditionalists, reservation dwellers, activists, etc.)? Do they say these people don't want me to learn this because I'm not Indian? Do they say they are fulfilling a prophecy supposedly made in the 1960s to teach Indian faiths to non-Indians despite protests by other Indians? If they tell you to avoid "real" Indians, they are doing it to protect their profits (not their prophets!). They know what Traditionalists and others will tell you about the falsity of this charade and the palpable damage it is doing to our communities. Yes, it is possible to learn these ways without being a Native, and non-Indians have done so for five centuries. However, it takes a lifetime of commitment shown in very mundane ways, and knowledge is not given simply because it is desired. This supposed prophecy may be based on prophecies revealed earlier regarding the intrinsic need for the coexistence of Indian and non-Indian religions, but you can bet that Unehlanvhi, Wakan Tanka, Yusin, Gitchi Manitou, nor any of the other manifestations of our Creator called for payment to be asked, other Indians to be excluded, or knowledge to be given before dedication has been proven.

Finally, as a feminist, you must ask yourself if you have been told that men and women should participate in all rituals together, regardless of the time of month or year. When you found out that traditional rites were often segregated and women were not active participants in some rituals in the case of menstruation, pre- or post-parturition, or seasonal cycle, were you told that the inclusiveness of New Age rituals strikes down the inherently sexist nature of the Old Ways? Given such misinformation, I cannot fault you for drawing the conclusion that New Age ceremonies are "improved" versions of older, exclusionary ones and therefore outside the purview of us benighted sisters who still hold to them. I cannot find fault with you for the same reason I cannot criticize the diction of a two-year-old, just learning to speak as an adult does. Have they told you that we did not take part in rituals during Moontime or when babies were due-or-new because we already possessed the benefits that the rituals granted other members of the community? Did they explain that the sometimes-segregation of Indian rites translated into community power for Native women, a power that was usurped by forced religious inactivity of women after Christian conversion?

A further admonition is to be wary of amalgamations. If you truly seek to follow a Native path, there are ways to do so. They will no doubt involve years of study with one or another holy person, probably in site-specific ceremonies (chain motels are never part of this repertoire, nor are lodges-for-hire in the hinterlands). This will probably be initiated only after you have sufficiently proven your diligence by acting as driver-on-a-moment's-notice for the holy person, often supplementing their grocery and cigarette fund from your own pocket, and after making the round of endless visits with family, friends, and powwow buddies, without ever being introduced or accorded any honor for your obvious culturally sensitive outreach efforts. If, after many years of this, you can accept with equanimity the fact that you may be told to "Get lost! No Indian wisdom for you here!," then you have walked the path to Traditionalism many of us have walked. It is easy to see the sort of dedication this requires and how the building of commitment/self-esteem in such endeavors can be the most valuable recovery vehicle available to Native women in crisis.

> Beyond the sexist strife, some East Coast worshipers have problems with the magical Native American branch of the (Goddess) movement. "The shamanistic tradition isn't the Goddess movement," says one New Jersey woman. "Some women are very adamant about not participating in Native American rituals, and now the Native American followers are pissed off. But the medicine wheel is not our symbol. Herbal healing is our tradition as North American witches." (She admits, however, that she and her friends "*have* done sweat lodges.") (Unger, 1990, p. 43)

If you cannot personalize the dilemma I present and care enough for your recovering sisters to allow them something all their own from which to derive strength, think of the position in which you may be placing yourselves. If you truly believe in indigenous peoples' principles, then you must be willing to accept the responsibility of carrying out the rituals or obligations of the faith to which you are inheritor. By respecting my sisters and I in our right to our faiths, perhaps first as a recovery tool, but certainly later as the cornerstone of our world-view, you also play a very important part in the balance. Find the tradition of your people, or one which is not tied to ethnicity as ours are. We do not belittle other pagans, and we do not despise "world religions," as is often portrayed. We feel each one plays its part, but that it is not right to force one on the practitioner of another, nor is it correct to assume that another faith is "there for the taking." Remember the healing power of self-respect, a healing power which was taken from Native women through centuries of collusion between church and state. Do not fall prey to unexamined beliefs. Just because a person is, or purports to be, an Indian (and the title "shaman/ess" is a real red light to be noted) telling you the secrets of her/his "tribe," don't take it at face value. Don't say prayers in a language you don't understand; are you certain of what it is you are saying? Don't rush headlong for those things which would be cautionary posts if you saw them in an identified religious "cult."

The matter of religious imperialism for Native women (and men) is no longer a small problem, one which we failed to address years ago when its nascent ludicrousness was less widely-accepted by "progressives" in our country. There is a chance for *real* progress in Indian Country by returning to those traditions of old. Healthy Native women together can make headway in the recapturing of our old positions of respect in our communities, but not so long as many of us suffer the degradation of substance and/or personal abuse. We can recover our health by recovering our traditions, but only if they remain intact, and if you, our sisters, refuse to collude with our further disenfranchisement. If you do not see the wrongness of religious imperialism, I fear for future generations of all our people. Already, New Age pseudo-Indian beliefs are beginning to take on elements of physical, as well as psychological, imperialism. In an open letter to (the now deceased) SunBear/Napoleon LaDuke in the Early Summer 1988 edition of *Akwesasne Notes*, Austrian doctor/shaman-watcher Roman Schweidlenka says that some plastic medicine men/women are becoming increasingly paranoid as they are challenged to authenticate their synthetic systems of belief. He says that, in particular, Harley Swift Deer has confederated with ultra-right occult practitioners, likening them to the occultists of the Third Reich. Schweidlenka quotes Swift Deer:

> . . . traditional Indians have race hatred and have to die out according to the Great Spirit's plan, because they do not fit into the new time, the New Age. (Spektor, 1989, p. 20)

Let us truly regard one another as sisters and respect each other's traditions without needing to own them. Let us offer our recovering sisters every vehicle by which to regain their health. Let us show true affinity by acting concertedly to keep the hearts of our women off the ground.

NOTE

1. "Indian Country" refers to the cultural, as well as the physical, "map" of indigenous communities in the United States. With more than one-half of all Natives living off the reservation, the cultural geography of Indian Country is more inclusive than the physical limits of Indian-owned land.

REFERENCES

Baudrillard, John (1975). *The mirror of production*. St. Louis, MO: TELOS Press.

Churchill, Ward (1992). *Fantasies of the master race: Literature, cinema and the colonization of American Indians*. Monroe, ME: Common Courage Press.

Collections of the South Carolina Indian Historical Society, vol. v (1897). Richmond: South Carolina Historical Society.

Crow Dog, Mary and Erdoes, Richard (1990). *Lakota woman*. New York: Grove Weidenfeld.

Magnuson, Jon (1989). Selling the Native American soul. *The Christian Century*, Nov. 22, 1084-7.

Spektor, Mordecai (1989). Shamans or charlatans? Do some teachers of Native American spirituality distort Indians' culture? *Utne Reader, July/August*, 15, 18, 20.

Unger, Rusty (1990). Oh, goddess! Feminists and witches create a new religion from ancient myths and magic. *New York*, June 4, pp 40-6.

Altared States:
Lesbian Altarmaking
and the Transformation of Self

Patricia Gargaetas

SUMMARY. Despite the changes in women's social and economic roles which are altering the way many women view themselves and the world in which they live, American society and popular culture provide few models and acceptable symbols from which women can gain energy and power. Phyllis Chesler (1989) says, "For women to imagine and honor a female deity is a sign of mental health" (p. xx). This paper investigates the choices of symbols employed on lesbians' home altars and the uses to which the altars are put. By selecting symbols intelligible to themselves, investing those symbols with import and intent, and using them on a home altar, these women are taking crucial steps in the transformation of Self.

Patricia Gargaetas (PGar) is a forty-five year old radical dyke who completed her Master of Arts in Anthropology at California State University, Sacramento in 1993. Lesbian altarmaking was the topic of her thesis, and women's spirituality continues as an ongoing subject of radically empiric research. She is currently committing culture under the propitious patronage and auspicious auspices of Silly Sisters' Art for the Millennia.

Address all correspondence to Patricia Gargaetas, 902 9th Avenue, Sacramento, CA 95818-4047.

[Haworth co-indexing entry note]: "Altared States: Lesbian Altarmaking and the Transformation of Self." Gargaetas, Patricia. Co-published simultaneously in *Women & Therapy* (The Haworth Press, Inc.) Vol. 16, No. 2/3, 1995, pp. 95-105; and: *Women's Spirituality, Women's Lives* (ed: Judith Ochshorn, and Ellen Cole) The Haworth Press, Inc., 1995, pp. 95-105; and: *Women's Spirituality, Women's Lives* (ed: Judith Ochshorn, and Ellen Cole) Harrington Park Press, an imprint of The Haworth Press, Inc., 1995, pp. 95-105. Multiple copies of this article/chapter may be purchased from The Haworth Document Delivery Center [1-800-3-HAWORTH; 9:00 a.m. - 5:00 p.m. (EST)].

95

"For feminist thinkers of the present era
the first and most fundamental act of our own emancipation
was granting ourselves authority as perceivers."
(Frye, Marilyn, 1992, p. 61)

As may be true of any interesting and complex topic, the subject of personal home altars has become a nexus, a point which connects a continuous outpouring of information and energy as well as a point at which to create a locus from which to perceive the context as it forms. My analysis is influenced more by my location at this point of continuously outpouring energy and information than by a location within disciplinary boundaries. In my work, I draw from the litera- ture of anthropology, as well as from the praxis of fieldwork–the received text and methodology of the craft of anthropology. In addi- tion, I draw from women's (not gender) studies, religious studies, feminist analyses and lesbian philosophies, and the academic as well as the nonacademic literature of feminist spirituality. I have become an observer/participant/perceiver, avoiding constraint by any analyti- cal focus constructed to conform to disciplinary boundaries. Although this work is grounded in radical feminist anthropology, I do not confine myself to radicalism, feminism, or anthropology.

I began my study with an observation: Women–lesbians in par- ticular–are making altars in their homes. My initial questions origi- nate in informal observation of altars in the homes of lesbians of my acquaintance. Altars were, even in my own home, implicit objects, unquestioned parts of the scenery. In this paper, I present an explication of the meaning of altar objects and altar work as described by participants and locate lesbian altarmakers[1] within a context of personal transformation and conscious ritual for change. My stance toward the women who have participated is both reflex- ive and dialogic; dialogue is by nature interactive. As can be expected, the participants have had an influence on my understand- ing of personal home altars; the project itself has also had an effect on individual altarmakers, myself included.

I focus my study on lesbians, although I found no significant differences of intent in altars created by lesbians, bisexuals, or het- erosexuals who participated. Regardless, as a lesbian, I choose to attend to lesbian existence. In *Compulsory Heterosexuality and Les-*

bian Existence, her ground-breaking essay in lesbian feminist theory, Adrienne Rich (1980) defines the term *lesbian existence* by saying, "[T]he word lesbianism has a clinical and limiting ring. Lesbian existence suggests both the fact of the historical presence of lesbians and our continuing creation of the meaning of that existence" (p. 20). Not only does Rich point to "[t]he virtual or total neglect of lesbian existence," she asserts, "Any theory or cultural/political creation that treats lesbian existence as marginal . . . is profoundly weakened thereby, whatever its other contributions" (p. 4).

In lesbian existence, how, and in what direction, a woman focuses her attention are philosophical, political and spiritual choices. Lesbian philosopher Sarah Lucia Hoagland (1988) says, "That I attend certain things and not others, that I focus here and not there, is part of how I create value" (pp. 91-92). Through altarmaking–a form of spiritual, political and philosophical attention–women willfully create value. Philosophical sister Marilyn Frye (1992) notes Hoagland's presentation of "lesbian community as a partly deliberate project of creating value, as opposed to just aligning ourselves with or against values in a preexisting scheme of value" (p. 26). Altar work engages will in the making of value.

Kay Turner (1990) describes an altar as "a sacred space set apart for the perpetuation and validation of an empowering discourse . . . that upholds and promotes . . . spiritual and ethical ideals" (p. 450). Although altarmakers in this study are not expressing the same heritage as the *altaristas* Turner treats in her doctoral dissertation, *Mexican American Women's Home Altars: The Art of Relationship*, her definition of altar holds.[2] Of *altarista*, Turner (1990) also observes:

> On the altar holy images are combined and recombined during the course of a woman's life. The same saints or representations of the Virgin may have different meanings to different women. Conventional or received meanings are altered, reconstituted, or transformed according to the individual histories, experiences, and preferences of the women. (p. 170)

This process is not unlike that of these lesbian altarmakers who have, perhaps, taken it one step further by not requiring the sharing of content and form *or* of received meaning. It is the *process* of altarmaking, rather than conventions of form or content, that is relevant to these altarmakers and their altars. As Naomi Goldenberg (1979) says in her foundational work, *The Changing of the Gods: Feminism and the Death of Traditional Religions,* "I am going to argue that it is not necessary. . . to share the *same* myths, images, and symbols. Instead, it is more important . . . [to] share the *process* of symbol creation itself" (p. 53).

These altars can be described and categorized as ones which exhibit an eclectic profusion or appear restrained by the orthodoxy of a ritual tradition (more profuse than orthodox). These altarmakers are neither adhering to nor creating sets of rules for correct construction, acceptable objects, or proper placement. Altars are ephemeral, as one participant emphasized at the end of the interview, "That is the altar *this* week," implying it will change (A-10).[3] Altars are in motion. An altarmaker reports:

> It is very hard to confine them. There is an interdigitation between what is part of the altar and what is not part of the altar . . . Things slop out into other spaces, and things encroach into the space. [The] shape of the altar . . . changes. It grows. It shrinks. It sends out pseudopods. (A-2)

A woman explicitly states: "The contents of altars are constantly changing" (Q-17). One says, "Altars . . . keep changing, with the seasons, with personal circumstances, for the sake of change" (Q-11). Another says, "This is a working altar. Objects change, are handled and moved about as the spirit moves me/them" (Q-30). Women use altars to move their lives. A participant says she began "relating the altar to [her] own internal seasons, and noticed movement . . . that reflected things that were going on for [her] emotionally and physically" (A-1). She says,

> My participation with my altar is something I have never been able to force. When the time came . . . it always just came to me. When I have tried to move [the altar] around without that feeling, I couldn't do it for very long; it didn't happen. (A-1)

Philosophically, she adds, "Soon things will change, and the altar will change" (A-1). Rather than using a formula with specific components combined in a specific manner, these altars tend to be more the result of recipes passed hand-to-hand, improvised, expanded and contracted to suit the need and the available ingredients.

Personal home altars are exceptional media for developing a recipe for a spirituality of one's own, a spirituality centered in (but not necessarily on) the Self.[4] In *The Spiritual Significance of the Self-Identified Woman*, Elsa Gidlow (1981) uses the term *self-identified* to describe those "[t]houghtful women who have come to realize that we must seek . . . . our spiritual path guided by our own inner light" (p. 74). Personal home altars kindle and feed such lights. Gidlow (1981) begins with the premise that "spiritual power grows from a ground of personal wholeness," that we are born "as . . . whole being[s]," but that if "the inner sense of wholeness is lost or discouraged from maturing, the individual becomes maimed and susceptible to indoctrination, manipulation and mastery" (p. 73). Phyllis Chesler (1989) asserts: "For women to imagine and honor a female deity is a sign of mental health" (p. xx). Altar work is a transformative act which engenders personal wholeness, is certainly beneficial to women's mental health, and is a self-identified aspect of women's culture.[5] One woman has what she describes as traditional tools on her altar–an altar cloth, a censer, an athame (ritual knife), a cup, a pentagram, Goddess icons, and sacred jewelry. These items, along with candlesticks and a mirror–either clear, to acknowledge divinity or self-worth, or black, for scrying (divination)–are always on her altar; however, numerous other items appear, depending on work she is doing at the altar. They can include her own initiating cords, articles from spells in progress, photographs of herself or others with whom she is concerned, favorite sayings, notes from friends, and various elemental and natural objects such as stones, crystals, feathers, salt, oil, flowers, bones, and fur. She says, "Over the years I have put all sorts of things on altars. I can usually find a rationale to use just about anything that takes my fancy" (Q-26).

Altarmaking is a cognitive as well as an intuitive act, discerning and full of discriminating awareness. It is a product of cognition in the broad sense that it includes both awareness and judgment, rather than in the limited sense that it is necessarily based on or even capable of being reduced to empirical facts. The great variety of objects chosen by altarmakers reflect their experiences and desires as well as the symbol systems those experiences and desires render intelligible; however, personal home altars are not phenomenal; they express both conscious thought and intuition. An altar is also an embodiment *and* a manifestation of an altarmaker and her intent, although many of the symbols through which that intent is embodied and manifested are eclectic and variable. Even when arising out of a specific ritual tradition, in many cases symbols are explicable only by the altarmaker. For the altarmaker, working an altar can be what symbolic anthropologist Barbara Myerhoff (1990) defines as *emergent ritual*–ritual which need not "cluster about a set of shared, powerful and axiomatic symbols" (p. 248).

An altar is a location at which the Self displays itSelf, as well as a place where conscious change can be set in motion. One altarmaker says, "At times I activate my altar by lighting a candle. . . . Other times I wave my hand over it and ask the energies to rise" (A-8). An altarmaker works her altar by focusing her intent, expressing her will, her desire, herSelf. She meditates. She prays. She activates images and changes her attitudes. Visibly, palpably, she creates a mental realm and an emotional locus in which connections can be effected, transformations actuated and identity consciously be altered. In discussing the transformation of consciousness in ritual, Barbara Myerhoff (1990) says,

> A transformation is a major and lasting change: in structure, appearance, character or function. One becomes something else, . . . One has an altered state of consciousness, a new perception of oneself or one's socio/physical world, a conversion in awareness, belief, sentiment, knowledge, understanding; a revised and enduring emergent state of mind and emotion. (p. 245)

Women give meditation, centering, and focusing all as reasons to have an altar and as altar activities. They aptly articulate this aspect of altarmaking: "I wanted a way to symbolize my internal state and ongoing spiritual process" (Q-33); "I wanted a symbolic and visual representation of my feeling that my life was becoming sacred, or at least that I was experiencing it as sacred"

(Q-31); "I wanted to focus and draw better energy into my life" (Q-19); "I use my altar to help me meditate" (Q-15); "I was taking gigantic steps in my life with much risk. I frequently needed a way to center, a way to release fear and create energy" (Q-14); "Creating and tending the altar . . . is very necessary to my spiritual equilibrium" (Q-11); "I felt the need to learn how to create some peace in my life" (Q-9); "I needed to create the space and time to get to know and create a relationship with myself. Allowing my energy to express itself in the form of an altar facilitated the process" (Q-6).

The women elucidate further: "On my altar I have bundles consisting of shells, stones, and crystals in various combination wrapped in a ti leaf. These are something I make to focus energy on a particular intention . . . " (Q-30). "I reactivate my altar as my focus in life changes, intensifies, or expands" (Q-25); "Despite my best efforts, 'God' still surreptitiously visits me as an old bald bearded man on a cloud. I hope the altar will exorcise him as it exalts the Goddess in her various guises" (Q-22); "I first built an altar to my child self. I was in a painful struggle with my family and built an altar to heal the rift" (Q-8); "I was seeking some balance and peace in my life that I could not find in the context of the religion in which I was raised" (Q-4); "I performed a simple ritual symbolizing my sorrow, frustration" (Q-3); "My altar is ripe with possibilities, reminders, and warnings" (Q-2).

One woman says, "I need a lot of dyke-positive symbols on my altar and in my home to counteract the hateful messages of the world" (Q-16). For many women, part of coming out as a lesbian involves living alone or having a space of her own, sometimes for the first time in her life. As one participant declares, "First I needed my own home" (Q-28). An altarmaker comments,

> I clearly remember when it became *real* important for me to set up an altar. It was when I rented a cottage for the express purpose of making art, and also to have my own space. I had two teenagers at the time, and I was still married, and I really needed my own space. . . . I had two little rooms, and I took the door off and I put it on supports, and consciously made an altar. I did the four directions. I incorporated symbols for the

Earth, the Water, the Fire, the Air. It was much more of a traditional, formalized altar. (A-6)

Another elaborates,

There is an aspect of the altars that has to do with *having* a place which is your own in which it can be established. Having a place which you claim as your own is important. Even though the house is supposed to be a woman's domain, it has not been women's space. In women's space, in the spirit of Virginia Woolf's *A Room of One's Own*, women now say, "This is an altar. I say this is an altar. This is sacred space. This is where I focus. Here is where I attend." (A-10)

Having money and a room of one's own–economic and emotional resources–are aspects which help give lesbian altarmakers the ability to attend, which, as noted previously, gives a woman focus for her philosophical, political and spiritual choices.

Altars are symbolic expressions of women's culture, a spiritual art form–ephemeral by nature–of personal transformation and conscious change. On her personal home altar, a woman seizes power, the power inherent in symbols, the power of individual action to change the world beginning with herSelf. Barbara Myerhoff (1982) makes constructive commentary on useful methods to effect such transformation: "We have to develop rituals and employ symbols in increasingly private contexts, living as we do in a diffuse, fragmented world with shattered or shallow consensual structures" (p. 126). This is precisely what altarmakers are doing, forming concepts of the sacred using anything symbolic and meaningful in their own experience (Q-16).

As noted earlier, personal home altars make the Self visible to itSelf, a concept I correlate with Barbara Myerhoff's (1986) analysis in her work with elderly Jewish immigrants in Venice, California. "By denying their invisibility, isolation, and impotence, they [make] themselves be seen, and in being seen they [come] into being in their own terms, as authors of themselves" (p. 263). As Mary Daly (1978) declares, "The strength which Self-centering women find . . . is our *own* strength. . . . used by women who name the sacred on our own authority. . . . women who choose to be our own authors, authoring our Selves" (p. 49).

Altarmakers are neither waiting for others to create the shape of the future nor permitting others to define the symbols which empower action and transform the Self. Structures constructed through the patriarchal institutions of the majority culture do not give impetus to the changes required for a transition from a patriarchal paradigm. Women have been, as Barbara Myerhoff (1982) also says, "left to devise for ourselves the myths, rituals, and symbols needed to endow life with clarity and significance" (p. 129). For altarmakers, the results of being left to their own devices are prodigious. They have literally taken matters into their own hands and are–as Myerhoff (1982) predicted would be the result of such action–doing a decent job. In discussing ritual and symbol as a form of self-creation, Myerhoff (1982) also says, "the realization that one can and should begin to play with ritual symbols and enact their truths, is the first and hardest step [in transformation]" (p. 131). These altarmakers have taken that first and most difficult step by creating and activating symbols intelligible to themselves and investing those symbols with import and intent. As phrased by one altarmaker,

> We are exploring, not trying to do things perfectly . . . Women have had responsibility without power, have been in charge of the random elements of society. Women have a keen appreciation of the inability to do anything perfectly. If something feels right we keep doing it. What is important is not that it be done perfectly, but that it be done. (A-2)

NOTES

1. Throughout this work I use Kay Turner's term *altarmaker* and its logical extrapolations to refer to the women who construct and work altars. In an endnote to the first chapter of her doctoral dissertation, *Mexican-American Women's Home Altars: The Art of Relationship*, Turner (1990) traces her use of the terms *altarista* and *altaristas* (altarmaker–singular and plural) to personal communication with "Chicana artist Amalia Mesa Baines, who learned the domestic altar tradition from women in her family." Turner reports, "The designation was readily understood by my consultants and integrated into our conversations, so I have taken the liberty of using it throughout the text" (p. 53).

2. Like Kay Turner (1990), I think "[t]he history of Western women's creation and maintenance of the domestic altars requires a full length study" (p.

53). In a seven page footnote in her doctoral dissertation, *Mexican-American Women's Home Altars: The Art of Relationship,* Turner (1990) provides a brief historical summary from which she concludes that "further research would most likely recover evidence to support my sense that the Western domestic altar tradition has been carried forth over millennia, from the deep past up to the present" (p. 54).

3. Throughout this work, I use the designations Q-(plus a number) and A-(plus a number) to cite participants in the Women's Altar Project. The designation *Q* is for participants who filled out a questionnaire, while *A* is used for participants I interviewed and whose altars I photographed. In addition to the traditional anthropological research method of participant observation, I also used visual anthropology (I photographed altars), radical empiricism (I made altars), oral interviews and narrative questionnaires. Using a snowball technique, I conducted ten interviews in Sacramento, California, between September and December, 1990. I secured questionnaires through an advertisement in the August/September (1992) issue of *Lesbian Connection: A Nationwide Forum of News & Ideas for, by and About Lesbians* (A Publication of the Helen Diner Memorial Women's Center & Ambitious Amazons, Elsie Publishing Institute, P.O. Box 811, East Lansing, MI 48826). Like the snowball technique I used to locate women who were willing to be interviewed and have their altars photographed, the responses to the advertisement in no sense constitute a random sample. In all cases, the women selected themselves by their willingness to participate. The return rate for the questionnaires requested via the advertisement was excellent; of forty-six requested, thirty-two were returned (almost 70 percent). These women represent a minuscule percentage of the women who subscribed to, purchased, or read one of the 21,000 copies printed in this particular issue of *Lesbian Connection.* I could only speculate about how many of those women are altarmakers or how many who are altarmakers actually responded. However, the information from the questionnaires is in accord with and supports the information gathered in the interviews I conducted locally.

4. The term *mySelf* appears in the questionnaire material in response to the question, "Do you have a spiritual or religious affiliation?" As defined by Mary Daly (1987):

Self [first appeared in *Gyn/Ecology: The Metaethics of Radical Feminism.* Boston: Beacon Press, 1978] *n*: the Original core of one's own be-ing that cannot be contained within the State of Possession [patriarchy]; living spirit/matter: the psyche that participates in Be-ing. (p. 95)

Self with the capital *S* extrapolates to words such as *mySelf, yourSelf, herSelf.*

5. Kay Turner (1990) says women's culture is "a culture distinct from but operating within the general culture . . ." (p. 33). Gerda Lerner (1986) says, "Women's culture is the ground upon which women stand in their resistance to patriarchal domination and their assertion of their own creativity in shaping society . . . It is important to understand that woman's culture is never a subculture . . ." (p. 242).

REFERENCES

Chesler, Phyllis. (1989). Foreword. In Z. Budapest. *The holy book of women's mysteries (Complete in one volume): Feminist witchcraft, goddess rituals, spellcasting, and other womanly arts* (pp. xix-xx). Oakland, CA: Wingbow Press.

Daly, Mary. (1978). *Gyn/Ecology: The metaethics of radical feminism.* Boston: Beacon Press.

Daly, Mary (Conjured in Cahoots with Jane Caputi). (1987). *Websters' first new intergalactic wickedary of the English language.* Boston: Beacon.

Frye, Marilyn. (1992). *Willful virgin: Essays in feminism 1976-1992.* Freedom, CA: Crossing Press.

Gidlow, Elsa. (1981). The spiritual significance of the self-identified woman. *Maenad. 1*(3), 73-79.

Goldenberg, Naomi R. (1979). *The changing of the gods: Feminism and the death of traditional religions.* Boston: Beacon Press.

Hoagland, Sarah Lucia. (1988). *Lesbian ethics: Toward new value.* Palo Alto, CA: Institute of Lesbian Studies.

Lerner, Gerda. (1986). *The creation of patriarchy.* New York: Oxford University Press.

Myerhoff, Barbara. (1982). Rites of passage: Process and paradox. In Victor Turner (Ed.), *Celebration: Studies in festivity and ritual* (pp. 109-135). Washington, DC: Smithsonian Institution Press.

Myerhoff, Barbara. (1986). Life not death in Venice: Its second life. In Victor Turner & Edward M. Bruner (Eds.), *The anthropology of experience* (pp. 261-286). Urbana, IL: University of Illinois Press.

Myerhoff, Barbara. (1990). The transformation of consciousness in ritual performances: Some thoughts and questions. In Richard Schechner & Willa Appel (Eds.), *By means of performance: Intercultural studies of theatre and ritual* (pp. 245-249). Cambridge: Cambridge University Press.

Rich, Adrienne. (1980). *Compulsory heterosexuality and lesbian existence.* Denver: Antelope Publications.

Turner, Kay Frances. (1990). *Mexican-American women's home altars: The art of relationship.* Unpublished doctoral dissertation, University of Texas, Austin. (University Microfilms No. 9031732).

Liberating the Amazon:
Feminism and the Martial Arts

Sharon R. Guthrie

SUMMARY. In this paper, I challenge the Cartesian emphasis on mind that characterizes much of feminist theory and propose instead a feminist "care of the self" ethics that revolutionizes both mind and body. Qualitative research involving participant-observation and 30 indepth interviews with women who practice seido karate at Thousand Waves, a feminist martial arts dojo in Chicago, provide empirical support for such a proposition. Data indicated that women's self concept is profoundly altered when physically empowering activities such as the martial arts are practiced in gynocentric spaces infused with feminist spirit, ethics, and pedagogy. They also indicated that healing from incest, rape and other forms of violence is facilitated by martial arts/self defense training in ways that are qualitatively different from traditional psychological therapy. Ultimately, this work suggests that approaches that empower women physically, as well as mentally and spiritually, may be more effective in producing personal and social change than cognitive strategies alone.

Sharon R. Guthrie, PhD, Physical Education from The Ohio State University, Assistant Professor (psycho-social specialist), Department of Physical Education, California State University, Long Beach; Co-editor: *Women and Sport: Interdisciplinary Perspectives* (forthcoming, Human Kinetics Publishers, 1994); affiliations: NWSA (National Women's Studies Association), AAHPERD (American Alliance of Health, Physical Education, Recreation & Dance), NASSS (North American Society for Study of Sport Sociology); address: 1250 Bellflower Boulevard, Long Beach, CA 90840.

[Haworth co-indexing entry note]: "Liberating the Amazon: Feminism and the Martial Arts." Guthrie, Sharon R. Co-published simultaneously in *Women & Therapy* (The Haworth Press, Inc.) Vol. 16, No. 2/3, 1995, pp. 107-119; and: *Women's Spirituality, Women's Lives* (ed: Judith Ochshorn, and Ellen Cole) The Haworth Press, Inc., 1995, pp. 107-119; and: *Women's Spirituality, Women's Lives* (ed: Judith Ochshorn, and Ellen Cole) Harrington Park Press, an imprint of The Haworth Press, Inc., 1995, pp. 107-119. Multiple copies of this article/chapter may be purchased from The Haworth Document Delivery Center [1-800-3-HAWORTH; 9:00 a.m. - 5:00 p.m. (EST)].

Reclaiming female identity, which has been defined and controlled by male scientists, physicians, psychiatrists, and theologians, is one of the significant agendas of feminism. In this paper, I examine a mind/body/spiritual practice that contributes to women's agency, self determination, and healing through what is referred to as a feminist "care of the self" ethic. The need for such an ethic is premised on my belief that gender identity, that is, the ideological construction of feminine and masculine, constitutes the dominant and repressive form of self identification in western societies. Feminists have argued that such ideology is particularly oppressive to women because it is derived from Cartesian dualism, which labels the body as inferior to the mind and then associates bodily functions with females and mental functions with males. Although feminists have developed alternative theories and images of female identity, they emphasize primarily the intellectual dimension in promoting social change. Ironically, their intellectual focus, albeit on the reconstruction of patriarchal societies and female identity, perpetuates Cartesian dualism. It also contributes to an insufficient awareness that gender construction, which involves male control and oppression of female bodies, is ultimately rooted in the threat and practice of male violence against women. Indeed, Bart (1979), and Bart and O'Brien (1993) have argued that rape is the paradigmatic practice of our sexist society.

THEORETICAL BACKGROUND

The work and death of Mary Jo Frug, a feminist law professor, who was slashed to death on a street in Cambridge, Massachusetts, provides a startling example of the role violence and femicide play in controlling women, even those who are cognitively empowered. In her posthumously published draft (1992), she discusses the meaning of the female body and claims that legal rules permit and sometimes mandate:

> . . . the terrorization of the female body. This occurs by a combination of provisions that inadequately protect women against physical abuse and that encourage women to seek refuge against insecurity. One meaning of the "female body,"

then, is a body that is "in terror," a body that has learned to scurry, to cringe, and to submit. (pp. 1049-1050)

I agree with Frug's contention that terrorization of the female body by men is a problem common in patriarchal societies and is largely socially constructed. Frug, however, sought changes in legal rules in order to end this terror, arguing that "only when the word 'woman' cannot be coherently understood, will oppression by sex be fatally undermined" (p. 1075). In contrast, I do not believe that this form of oppression will be eradicated with legal changes alone. Too often women are socialized to embody a disabling movement vocabulary as part of their feminine identity, that is, one emphasizing softness, vulnerability, physical weakness, and fear of injury. Successful resistance, therefore, requires a reconstruction of female identity that involves not only changes in the intellectual component of female socialization, but also the development of a physically empowered female self.

I refer to this process as feminist "care of the self"–a self-constitution of female identity that emphasizes the social construction of identity. This notion of care of the self is thus different from the concept of care associated with essentialist positions such as those of Nel Noddings. Noddings' (1986) ethical practice of caring, which is derived from women's "natural" mothering capacity, suggests the transformative ethical possibilities of an extension of self. Not only is her model deterministic and universal, it does not fully address whether women's moral response of caring is a function of their oppressed status. It also does not acknowledge the critical role violence against women plays in supporting such oppression. In contrast, empowered female identities, that is, multiple female subjectivities in continual and thoroughly contemplated processes of self creation, form the basis for my feminist care of the self ethic. Such an ethic is grounded in the following hypotheses: (1) care of the self must be embodied through mind/body practices, not just mental attitudes alone; (2) care of the self practices have a sociopolitical component and thus are not merely narcissistic; (3) resistance to gender oppression and a commitment to care of the self require developing a strong sense of self through practices that promote: (a) health and nutrition, (b) meditation, (c) physical strength and self defense skills, and (d) the study of feminist theory and strategies for successful resistance in group settings; and (4) such practices experienced in feminist spaces with feminist teachers committed to sexual equality can become the basis for developing empowering relationships with other women and collective structures capable of sustaining feminist goals and values.

RESEARCH METHODS AND SETTING

Such a feminist community and the practice of a feminist "care of the self" ethic is found at Thousand Waves, a martial arts dojo in Chicago for women only and children, both girls and boys. The dojo is owned and operated by two lesbian feminists who team teach approximately 160 students: 25% of them children, 10-16% women and children of color. This study was conducted during summer, 1993 using both indepth interviews and participant observation. Informants were 26 Caucasians and 4 women of color ranging in age from 26 to 62 years and in belt status from blue to black.

The primary martial art taught at Thousand Waves is seido karate. Like all forms of karate, seido karate is a kicking and punching art and thus develops self defense skills; however, seido also involves calm periods of meditation designed to enhance the focus and meaning of the movements. Moreover, to facilitate drawing upon one's inner reservoirs of energy (chi), aerobic activities, strength training, and a low fat, high fiber vegetarian diet are recommended. Therefore, although physical prowess is a product of training, seido karate is also a spiritual practice that fosters individual awareness and growth, as well as connections among mind, body and spirit and among self, others, and the universe.

Thousand Waves is not unique in emphasizing the spiritual foundation of the practice, although it is primarily dojos that follow Far Eastern traditions that include this important dimension. What does make Thousand Waves unique, however, is the feminist approach of the teachers who feel a strong sense of political mission, that is, they seek to reconstruct gender relations by creating an environment (community) that empowers women and girls and allows them to heal from the wounds inflicted by patriarchal oppression.

The teachers' commitment to achieving their feminist goals is demonstrated in numerous ways. First, the physical space, which was designed by a woman, is beautifully elegant, comfortable, and safe. Feminist touches are ubiquitous, including the presence of feminist art and literature, a locker room with a sauna, steamroom, and masseuse, and occasional meditation classes devoted to group discussion of feminist topics. Secondly, the teaching philosophy and methods emphasize self growth and cooperation with others, rather than competition and winning tournaments. Moreover, no woman is turned away because of race, size, or ability, and work study opportunities and scholarships are made available to those with financial difficulties. Thirdly, mentoring and bonding among members are strongly encouraged, as are social and political involvement in the community; for example, students demonstrate their martial art skills in the Gay Rights Parade and "take back the night" marches, and are actively involved in International Women's Day and the Chicago Women's Cancer Project.

Indeed, for most of the women, Thousand Waves serves as a feminist sanctuary where they may be fully authentic, escape the stressors of the patriarchal world, and associate with kindred spirits. All informants emphasized the importance of the gynocentric environment in promoting personal transformation. Not only do they prefer training in a woman only space, many believe that had their training begun in a male dominated dojo they would have quit. It is noteworthy, however, that these same women, who earlier would have quit, believe they now could train successfully in such a setting. Apparently, the attitudes and skills learned at Thousand Waves have empowered their perceptions of their abilities to mediate patriarchal environs.

FINDINGS

The findings of this work offer compelling evidence that women's embodiment, that is, the way they experience their bodies and minds, is profoundly altered by martial arts training at Thousand Waves. They also suggest the need to develop somatopsychic therapeutic models and approaches to women's mental health, rather than rely on those that do not recognize the critical role of the

body in attaining mental health and the social roots of mental illness. Findings supporting these claims are presented in the following section.

Empowerment

Empowerment of women–physical, mental, spiritual–is a central
goal at Thousand Waves. Indeed, all of the women interviewed
reported empowerment as one of the major benefits of martial arts
training. Although most were feminists prior to joining the dojo and
felt strengthened by their feminist ideologies, a significant majority
did not feel physically powerful. In fact, many had come to Thousand Waves for self defense training, hoping that such skills would
help them overcome their fears and sense of vulnerability.

A key factor making the Thousand Waves experience an empowering one is that the women learn to physically defend themselves.
More importantly, however, they learn they have the *right* to self
defend. As one woman remarked:

> What happens at Thousand Waves is the embodiment of fem-
> inist thought. That is, not only do we have the physical ability
> to defend ourselves, we also have the right to defend our-
> selves. This requires another level of acceptance, rooted in a
> valuing of the self which many women don't possess. The
> skills are worthless if you don't feel you have the right to
> defend yourself on the street, at home, or in the workplace.

Other factors fostering empowerment include the mental and spiritual challenges provided at Thousand Waves. One of the results of
meeting such challenges is an awareness of the importance of
persistence and spirit in achieving goals. As one woman com-
mented:

> The biggest lesson I have learned, that I apply to everything is:
> if you do something consistently over time, you get results and
> can reach your goals. It's part of the mind, body, spirit connec-
> tion: if strength meets technique, strength will win; however, if
> technique is matched with spirit, spirit will always conquer
> both strength and technique and find the way; the underlying
> message of Thousand Waves is you don't need great physical

strength or perfect technique, if you have strong spirit. Most of us wouldn't have lasted in any other school.

Using the image of a bonsai as a metaphor, one informant describes a common socialization experience for women in our culture, as well as how these experiences are deconstructed at Thousand Waves:

> Our strengths are pruned as is the bonsai, we become disabled. My mother found my tomboy instrumentalism embarrassing, so I shut down this aspect of myself. I did not develop discipline with anything and always felt ashamed of my independence and physical activity. Martial arts training at Thousand Waves enabled me to break through these self imposed boundaries and limits. I can see it in my personal life and at work. I have much more confidence.

Another recounts a similar process in a different way:

> I always felt fragile and fearful of harm. I thought that was how a woman was supposed to feel. The more fragile I felt, the more attractive I believed myself to be. Hence, I worked at this and was quick to turn my power over to others, particularly men. At Thousand Waves we gain a more accurate assessment of our bodily powers; as a result, we are able to shed warped notions of our own fragility, as well as other people's omnipotence. Martial arts has helped me break out of traditional feminine training and to recreate myself.

Closely related to a developing sense of empowerment, is an enhanced body image and awareness. All of the women expressed significant improvements in their perceptions of their bodies. Many were told as children that they were uncoordinated and clumsy, and thus developed no confidence in their motor skills. In the supportive, nonelitist environment of Thousand Waves, where the emphasis is on setting one's own standards rather than meeting universal norms, the informants gained an acceptance of and respect for their bodies:

> I was always trying to change my body. Before I focused a lot

on weight issues, continually dieting to control weight. Up and down, I felt like my body was out of control. I now have come to accept my body as it is and don't care as much what others think. I've learned to focus more on what it can do, rather than how it looks.

They also noted how improved body perception due to self defense training has resulted in changes in the way they posture and carry their bodies. Such changes have provided great benefits at work, in social settings, and particularly on the streets of Chicago:

There's been a big change in the way I posture my body. I call it 'posturing for power.' I don't have the same victim stance. I use my body differently than I did in the past and use space differently. Early on I noticed a drastic reduction in harassment on the street and in social settings. You start putting out confidence vibes and energy; it has a lot to do with changes, many times minute, in the body.

Although reductions in sexual harassment were commonly noted, an African American woman emphasized still another dimension of how martial arts training at Thousand Waves has changed her body image and carriage:

I have gotten rid of the posturing that represents the internalization of my own oppression. I now live in the Black community and don't focus on being more white. Blacks often denounce African features. I used to. Trying to be white is so metabolized for many of us, we usually don't stop to think about it. I have been able to stop this process at the bodily level and have really become proud of being Black. And it shows in the way I carry my body.

Healing

Healing is another significant theme emerging from the data. Many women at Thousand Waves are healing from incest, approximately 20% of our sample, while others are recovering from rape, eating disorders, drug abuse, and growing up in dysfunctional families. Although few of the women came to Thousand Waves for this specific purpose, healing has been a common result. The following quotes highlight the therapeutic gains derived from the Thousand Waves experience:

> The yelling aspect, e.g., the kiai, has been important for me. I have learned to use my voice and realized how my voice has been taken away from me. I have gotten rid of a lot of my anger as a result of martial arts training. Part of it is learning to center myself. Part of it is not feeling so helpless. I now feel as if I am taking care of myself.

> Fear was my issue, and my fear was stored in my body—stiffness, holding my breath were part of my way of being in the world. To break out of your fear pattern, you need to move physically. I have less fear now because I have developed stronger boundaries through my martial arts training; hence, I am not as fearful of relationships and intimacy. We become more conscious at Thousand Waves; consequently, repressed stuff comes up. It's not necessarily pleasant but is integral to the healing process.

Many of the women have been in therapy, and thus were able to compare benefits derived at Thousand Waves with those gained in traditional therapeutic settings. For them, karate as a mind-body discipline facilitates the healing process in ways that are compatible with, yet qualitatively different from, other psychological therapies:

> The martial arts is a type of physical and psychological therapy. I can go to karate and kick and punch through my feelings. I have also done therapy. Martial arts is not a replacement for talking therapy but what it does, that traditional therapy cannot do, is put you back in your body. I believe that my body remembers every thing that happened to it and that's why moving in karate helps in ways that are connected to say kicking and punching. Kicking and punching allow me access to my anger as a recovering alcoholic, as a child of alcoholics, and as a woman in our culture; martial arts at Thousand Waves allows me to express those feelings in a safe way; I suppose

you could do this in a therapist's office, punching a pillow, but this is sustained, long term healing that happens, particularly when you practice often.

I believe therapy and martial arts are complementary forms; I am now convinced, however, that ultimately healing has to come through the body; I think this is a shortcoming of traditional talking therapy. It makes perfect sense to involve the body because the pain is located in the body, it's not just in the head. Therapists often assume that healing is just some sort of mental process; the physical realm can open up for you what is not possible in purely mental therapy.

What happened to me as a child happened to my physical body. You cannot heal on a purely intellectual level, like what is emphasized in traditional therapy. Martial arts is a physically healing process. Feeling connected to your body is the first step to being connected to the rest of the world.

Martial Arts as Resistance

All of the informants believe that self defense is one of the most important survival skills a woman can possess. They also recognize that what they are learning at Thousand Waves is insurrectionary. Negative reactions from males (and sometimes females) to their martial arts training confirm their resistance. Central to this resistance is that women who can physically defend themselves are, in effect, neutralizing a significant power imbalance between females and males. As a result, most of the women perceive the activity as transformative socially, as well as personally:

What we are learning at Thousand Waves is absolutely radical. If women learn to defend themselves physically, you would see less sexual assault, fewer women willing to put up with being second class citizens and being abused. I see the body as the most fundamental level of dealing with patriarchy; intellectual theory is great; however, if that is the only thing I did I would be stuck in my head. We engage as physical beings in the world, thus I believe that we have to change the way we physically engage each other and the ways we communicate with each other, non-verbally and verbally. This is what I learn at Thousand Waves: new ways of communicating physically. I don't think you understand boundaries until you understand them at the physical level; you then can understand them at the emotional level. This is so important for women, because the physical level is the level that most of us are violated on.

One of the reasons men attack women physically is because they know women usually can't defend themselves. If there were a critical mass of Amazons out there who could physically challenge men's natural strength and force advantages, men would think twice before they moved into our spaces.

DISCUSSION AND CONCLUSIONS

These data provide strong evidence that female embodiment can be profoundly altered when physically empowering activities such as the martial arts are practiced in gynocentric spaces, particularly those that are infused with feminist spirit, ethics, and pedagogy. The findings also suggest that healing from incest, rape and other forms of violence is often facilitated by martial arts/self defense training and that such healing occurs in ways that are qualitatively different than traditional psychological therapy. It is clear, however, that the environment in which the martial arts are practiced, which includes the vision, ethics, methods, and qualities of those individuals who structure and participate in that environment, is a central element in maximizing such benefit.

Since the late 1960s, feminist martial artists and self defense teachers have emphasized self defense as a critical survival skill for women living in misogynist cultures. Others who have gathered extensive data on rape avoiders, most notably Pauline Bart and Patricia O'Brien (1993), have concluded that women who participate in sports, particularly contact sports, have a far better chance of avoiding physical assaults than those who are non-athletic. Despite the proliferating literature and research confirming that violence against women is pervasive, feminist liberation proposals have continued to emphasize mental rather than physical empowerment.

Although such strategies are an essential element in moving women forward politically, economically and socially, they have not eliminated the violence done to our bodies and minds, nor the deaths experienced by women such as Mary Jo Frug.

Similarly, psychotherapeutic models have tended to treat the client-patient as a disembodied entity (Pruzinsky, 1990), dismissing the importance of bodily experience in personality development and change. Important exceptions to this trend are therapists such as E. Sue Blume (1991) who has emphasized the importance of "body work" (e.g., massage, self defense) in facilitating recovery for incest survivors.

In order for feminism and therapy to be fully effective in empowering women, I believe they must include and integrate mind-body strategies. In this paper, I have tried to demonstrate how practices involving physical, mental, and spiritual empowerment of women may ultimately be more effective in transforming individuals and society than those that focus on cognitive activities alone. I refer to this model of transformation as a feminist care of the self ethic. Such an ethic offers women an alternative to constructing their identities in accordance with gender norms that associate femininity with vulnerability, physical weakness, and fear of injury. Women's successful resistance to these norms requires not only the shedding of an ideology of gender oppression and the development of a feminist perspective, but also the acquisition of gestures and movements associated with autonomy and physical empowerment.

Just as oppression is always embodied, a feminist care of the self ethic also must be embodied. This process is fostered by engaging in mind-body practices that develop a strong sense of self and emphasize: (a) health and nutrition, (b) meditation, (c) strength building and self defense training, (d) the study of feminist theory and strategies that effectively challenge gender stereotyping and oppression, and (e) discussion of study materials in group sessions. Such an ethic is further advanced by experiencing these mind-body practices in feminist spaces with feminist teachers. It is in such settings that feminist care of the self alternatives are most effective in developing empowered female identities at the individual level, as well as in facilitating the attainment of equality between women and men on broader social levels.

Thousand Waves provides strong evidence of such possibilities. In creating a feminist care of the self ethic, the community of women at Thousand Waves effectively challenges patriarchy at individual and small group levels. I also believe that their practices have deeper transformative potential. That is, although human transformation at Thousand Waves begins with the individual, the self constituting activities occur in a socio-political setting emphasizing feminist awareness and action, reciprocity in relationships, and service to the community. These results give me reason to believe that if a critical mass of females were exposed to this kind of environment and practice, particularly at young ages, we would see some drastic, and long awaited, changes in the way women experience not only their bodies but also their world.

REFERENCES

Bart, P. B. (1979). Rape as a paradigm of sexism in society. *Women's Studies International Quarterly, 2*(2), 347-357.

Bart, P. B., & O'Brien P. H. (1993). *Stopping rape: Successful survival strategies.* New York: Teachers College Press.

Blume, E.S. (1991). *Secret survivors: Uncovering incest and its aftereffects in women.* New York: Ballantine Books.

Frug, M. J. (1992). A postmodern feminist legal manifesto (An unfinished draft). *Harvard Law Review, 105*(5), 1045-1075.

Noddings, N. (1986). *Caring: A feminine approach to ethics and moral education.* Berkeley, CA: University of California Press.

Pruzinsky, T. (1990). Somatopsychic approaches to psychotherapy and personal growth. In T. F. Cash & T. Pruzinsky (Eds.), *Body images: Development, deviance, and change* (pp. 296-315). New York: The Guilford Press.

Feminist Wicca:
Paths to Empowerment

Lynda L. Warwick

SUMMARY. Women's spirituality has made available to women unique opportunities for empowerment. Feminist Wicca provides models of ways in which women can develop qualities traditionally denied women, provides teaching and role models within the Wiccan community for women to learn skills, and offers support and affirmation for lesbians as well as heterosexual women within a creative, woman-centered community. Wiccan perspectives provide a context within which to address such issues as violence against women, societal change, and environmental destruction. Feminist therapists who are aware of the resources offered by feminist Wicca can assist clients to develop positive identities as they manage identity development and disclosure.

Since the publication in 1979 of *Drawing Down the Moon*, Margot Adler's survey of Neo-Paganism and Wicca, the Neo-Pagan movement has become one of the fastest-growing forms of spirituality in this country. Some estimate that there are up to 200,000 members of this movement, which includes Neo-Pagans, Wiccans of various kinds, and people who are interested in exploring Native

Lynda Warwick, MA, is a doctoral candidate at Miami University.
Correspondence should be addressed to the author at the Psychology Department, Benton Hall, Miami University, Oxford, OH 45056.

[Haworth co-indexing entry note]: "Feminist Wicca: Paths to Empowerment." Warwick, Lynda L. Co-published simultaneously in *Women & Therapy* (The Haworth Press, Inc.) Vol. 16, No. 2/3, 1995, pp. 121-133; and: *Women's Spirituality, Women's Lives* (ed: Judith Ochshorn, and Ellen Cole) The Haworth Press, Inc., 1995, pp. 121-133; and: *Women's Spirituality, Women's Lives* (ed: Judith Ochshorn, and Ellen Cole) Harrington Park Press, an imprint of The Haworth Press, Inc., 1995, pp. 121-133. Multiple copies of this article/chapter may be purchased from The Haworth Document Delivery Center [1-800-3-HAWORTH; 9:00 a.m. - 5:00 p.m. (EST)].

American forms of spirituality. Neo-Paganism represents an eclectic collection of individuals and groups who celebrate varying forms of earth-based spirituality. Within these diverse groups there are resources available for the empowerment of women which have not been available through more traditional forms of spirituality. This paper will address ways in which a particular form of women's spirituality within the Neo-Pagan movement, feminist Wicca, offers resources to women that can potentially lead to improved self-image, increased range of skills, and connection with a strong, empowering community. In addition, I will provide resources for women who may be interested in reading further, will address ways in which the perspective of feminist Wicca can inform the work of feminist psychotherapy, and will discuss the process of identity formation as it applies to such groups as lesbians and Wiccans.

There are several forms of the Goddess-based spirituality known as Wicca, Witchcraft, or simply the Craft (Guiley, 1989). While there is no body of doctrine which all Wiccans share, most contemporary Wiccans use the term to mean a system of religious practice which includes worship of Goddess figures, observance of the pre-Christian Celtic agricultural calendar of festivals, and the practice of magic. Wicca as it is practiced in the United States and in Britain is largely a created tradition, although it derives inspiration from a variety of other pantheistic or polytheistic traditions. In America, people who identify as Wiccan can be loosely divided into traditional and non-traditional practitioners. Feminist Wicca, a non-traditional form, makes a feminist analysis of patriarchal oppression of women central to the practice of Goddess-oriented worship and magic. Important leaders in the feminist Wiccan tradition include Starhawk (i.e., 1979; 1987), whose work emphasizes eco-feminist, anti-nuclear, and human-rights oriented values; one of her goals is to offer men and women tools to change our culture into one that values and protects the environment and all living beings. Other leaders include Z. Budapest (1989), Diane Stein (1986; 1988), and Shekinah Mountainwater (1991), whose woman-only forms of feminist Wiccan practice focus on the empowerment of women in order to change the conditions of patriarchy under which women live. Unlike Starhawk, Z. Budapest explicitly supports the use of women's power to constrain men's ability to hurt women, and will not teach men about what she understands to be women's power until "the equality of the sexes shall be a reality" (Budapest, 1989, p. 3).

Feminist Wicca provides resources for women in several ways. First, the worship of goddess figures from many cultures provides powerful symbols of women's strength, creativity, and ability to wield power. Stories of god-figures, especially those based on the Stag King or the Green Man of ancient Britain, provide images of positive male power which is neither oppressive to women nor collusive in patriarchal abuses of power. Such models of masculinity can be useful both in feminist therapy with men and in individual men's work to participate less in the oppression of women (Ganley, 1988; Dienhart & Avis, 1991). Created or historically based images of cultures and mythology reflective of societies where women are held in respect are being developed by many feminist Wiccans, resulting in reinterpretations of patriarchal myths which are affirmative for both women and men. In addition, the feminist Wiccan community includes women who are active, powerful, expressive and instrumental, who are able to nurture themselves as well as others. Within the community, options exist for women to develop a variety of skills, those which are traditionally women's skills and those which are not.

Second, the Wiccan community is supportive of a wide variety of lifestyles and identities. Dianic Wicca, which includes only women, may represent the only form of religious practice which is particularly oriented toward lesbians and women's space. Feminist Wicca is often understood as the ongoing creation and discovery of women's mysteries, so all-women groups with woman-oriented celebratory and magical emphasis are common. All-women space can provide an atmosphere where survivors of male violence can work toward developing or reconnecting with a positive, sustaining sense of spirituality.

Third, the Wiccan community is highly creative. Rituals tend to be written or improvised for each celebration and may include aspects of theater, dance, art, poetry, singing, and creative ways of interacting among group members. Women can learn skills from others who are proficient at such arts and in turn can contribute to the well-being and learning of their teachers. The practice of magic requires that women learn attitudes of empowerment, of entitlement to having their needs met, and the ability to ask aloud for what they need and want. In many ways, feminist Wicca can be a path to empowerment for women.

Wicca provides powerful metaphors of ways that women can be in the world through the various characterizations of the Goddess. While feminist Jungians have long understood the power of Goddess archetypes, recent Jungian work such as that of Jean Bolen (1984) and Clarissa Pinkola Estes (1992) is now becoming recognized and assimilated by feminist Wicca. Within Wicca, the Goddess is understood as the triad of Maiden, Mother and Crone. Most goddess figures in mythology fit into at least one of those roles, and many encompass all three. Each aspect reflects different ways in which women can realize their potentials in the world. Goddess as Maiden is understood to be in charge of her own sexuality, active, strong, powerful, bonded with female companions, intelligent, assertive, and capable of play. The maiden is also the aspect of the Goddess which is intuitive, dark, magical, and associated with Mystery, many of the qualities which have been labeled dangerous and frightening by a patriarchal culture. Myths of Maiden goddess include those of Artemis, Diana, Persephone, Kore, and Athena, as well as those of the Amazons. As a woman works with the aspect of the Maiden, she becomes aware of her strengths, potentials, and abilities to know and understand herself. The Maiden represents women's right to own themselves, to be self-directed, and to have a wide variety of skills, talents, and competencies upon which to draw. Mountainwater (1991) points out that what she terms the Dark Maiden is often expressed in our culture as women who are taught to be passive, dependent, in need of male protection and without boundaries. In contrast, the assertive, joyful capacities represented by the Bright Maiden are often interpreted as women becoming pushy, aggressive, hard-boiled, superficial, and careless of other people. Positive expressions of the Maiden aspect include the ability to integrate the qualities of the dark Maiden, which include the capacity to be "surrendering, spontaneous, compassionate, gentle, subjective, intuitive and imaginative," with the qualities of the bright Maiden, which include the ability to be "strong, in control of her life, organized, disciplined, independent, objective, scientific and playful" (Mountainwater, 1991). Maiden images provide a context within which to understand the ways women are encouraged to behave within a patriarchal culture, while suggesting more enriching ways to use women's capabilities.

Goddess as Mother is often seen as empowered with traditionally feminine attributes, such as the ability to nurture, create, teach, and heal, as well as the ability to protect her children with ferocity. Mountainwater (1991) points out that six Mother powers, birthing, healing, nurturance, sexuality, organization and love, have either been taken from women by men, or have been relegated to "dirty work," which is work deemed suitable for women to do. In a similar vein, Adrienne Rich (1980) illustrates ways in which male power has been used to control women's sexuality, production, creativity, nurturance, and abilities to practice healing. Women working with Mother aspects can focus on empowering themselves through reclaiming the positive aspects of such powers, understanding how they have been transformed by patriarchal forces, and finding in them sources of strength, pride and direction. The power of the Mother aspect involves women's ability to connect with others in mutually intimate, sustaining, nurturing ways, which leads to the enhancement of self (Surrey, 1991). Mother aspect qualities are not necessarily associated with bearing and raising children, since women in feminist Wicca are valued whether or not they bear children, but can also suggest other kinds of enriching, deepening, creative and sustaining activities. Myths which address Mother goddesses include those of Demeter, Gaia, Kuan-Yin, Brigid, Aphrodite, and many others.

Goddess as Crone is understood to be an old woman, past childbearing age, who is wise, independent, capable of meeting her own needs or of sharing with others, and who is often associated with choice, change, death, transformation, and challenge. The symbol of the Crone survives in the caricature of the Halloween witch, who is old, ugly, and fearsomely powerful. Crone powers challenge the patriarchal notion that the best woman is one who is young, beautiful, a ready sexual and childbearing partner, and who has little wisdom or boundaries of her own. Women who work with the Crone aspect learn about hard choices, boundaries, endings, letting go, courage, the ability to be alone with themselves, and transformation. The Crone represents necessary destruction, as the counterpart of the Mother's generativity, and the ability to be differentiated within relationships. Myths of the Crone include those of Hecate, Kali-Ma, Cerridwen, and the Morrigan, goddess of battle.

Active, instrumental, expressive, and receptive qualities are all contained within the symbol of the Triple Goddess, and women can be empowered as they are encouraged to bring those qualities and abilities into their lives which are generally relegated to men in our culture. Women are able to incorporate these qualities without suffering a loss of connection with other women or with loved ones, because the dichotomization of male and female qualities, of expressive and instrumental, is seen as artificial. The ability to develop characteristics which are assigned to each of the Goddess aspects is seen as positive, and feminist Witches strive to develop a balance. In non-Dianic traditions, the God is seen as the model of what a non-oppressive man can be. He is not controlling, not possessive, is joyful and respectful and able to be both active and quiet. As the Green Man, the God willingly sacrifices himself for the good of the community, to allow the crops to grow as he is reborn. In such aspects as the Lord of the Wild Hunt (Celtic) and Dionysus (Greek), he is chaotic and powerful, but is not oppressive. In the rich mythology of feminist Wicca, men and women can find affirmation for discovering and deepening all aspects of themselves in their own process of healing and becoming empowered.

Within the Wiccan community, women encompass the full spectrum of roles. Women are leaders, teachers, healers, priestesses, herbalists, organizers, musicians, craftspeople, dancers, and magic makers. Women are warriors, activists, writers, poets, artists, financial managers and producers of newsletters and magazines. Women lead many of the pagan and Wiccan organizations and are public speakers for the movement. Women work within the legal system to protect and safeguard the right to religious freedom and to fight for Wiccans who are persecuted because of their religious beliefs. Women produce movies and cable television shows about Wicca, organize large public rituals, teach classes through community colleges, write books, produce tapes, and often maintain an intensive student load. Within Wicca, women are assumed to have talents, skills, something to say and the ability to say it.

The Wiccan community offers the opportunity for developing

strong relational connections, a source of strength as women's friendships have always been. Successful development of covens, or Wiccan work and worship groups, requires members to work toward developing a fairly high level of interpersonal skill, including the ability to nurture and to ask for and receive support, the ability to communicate clearly and to assume leadership, the commitment to building and maintaining strong relationships, and the willingness to value emotional intimacy. Because it is difficult to hold a coven together in the face of many personalities accustomed to patriarchal values, members of a group which manages to work through the issues raised by being an emotionally intense, intimate group can emerge with a great deal of growth and learning. In addition, identifying as a Witch is an act of resistance in a culture which is Judeo-Christian, and the process of actively resisting patriarchal cultural norms can lead to growth and empowerment.

Feminist Wicca provides a forum in which lesbians and, less often, gay men, can find a spiritual environment which goes beyond "acceptance" or "tolerance" to affirmation and celebration. While the focus of traditional Wicca on male-female polarity is less appealing to many gay or lesbian witches, non-traditional Wicca focuses less on polarity and more on other means of addressing the sacred. Thus, lesbians can work within all-women or all-lesbian groups, focus on the Triple Goddess, and avoid the vocal or silent censure often faced in other religious traditions. Gay men occasionally form "faerie" covens, although this seems to be uncommon. Even in mixed groups, the celebration of women through Goddess worship tends to make the heterosexual norms of our society less salient and, depending on the makeup of particular groups, can lead to a powerfully affirming environment for gay and lesbian members. While members of individual groups will need to confront their homophobia, the ethic within feminist Wicca is that any form of non-exploitative, responsible sexuality is acceptable and that gay men and lesbians can provide new ways of participating in the Mystery.

Finally, feminist Wicca maintains an ethic of care for members of the community as well as for the environment. The emphasis is on coexistence and pluralism rather than on the control and exploitation of those who are different from some imagined norm, and the overall world view focuses on healing and changing what is wrong with the world and with individuals and on celebrating a life-affirming perspective. Wiccan theology is not thanophobic, since it sees death as an essential and intrinsic part of life, and this perspective allows for a long-range perspective on social and environmental issues. Many Wiccans believe either literally or symbolically in reincarnation and in karma, the notion that present action impacts future experience in a one-to-one positive or negative correspondence. This can make it difficult to "pass the buck" for such issues as environmental destruction or the cycle of poverty onto the next generation; believing that one might somehow return to the unsolved problems in the future is a good weapon against denial and indifference. There is a strong ethic that each person take personal responsibility for his or her actions. Wiccans are bound by the Wiccan Rede, which states, "An it harm none, do what you will." "None" is assumed to include self, and the Rede forbids exploitative or manipulative attempts to better one's situation. Wiccans are expected to work on their personal issues, to face and work to heal their wounds, to learn the faces of the deities which guide their struggles, and receive support for doing so from teachers or from their coven. Feminist Wiccans tend to emphasize both the power of the individual and of the group to effect change, while trying to avoid the New Age concept which suggests that individuals wholly create their own reality and therefore "choose" to live in oppressive, degrading, painful circumstances for the purposes of personal growth. Becoming able to take responsibility for taking care of self as well as others is a catalyst for change for many women, who are used to meeting the needs of others first and often to the exclusion of their own needs.

While feminist Wicca struggles to keep feminist values central in the development of its practice, the extent to which the movement as a whole succeeds in demonstrating feminist ideals varies. As a movement, contemporary Wicca tends to be somewhat racist and classist; most practitioners are well-educated middle-class white people with the luxury to address issues of personal growth and meaning in their lives. Unlike traditional Wicca, feminist Wicca is more a literary than an oral tradition, and the books and paraphernalia can be expensive to accumulate. Attending festivals or intensive training classes, which is often a primary way to gain skills, experience, and to make contacts, is also expensive and requires flexibility to take several days or a week off work. In addition, the tendency of non-traditional Wicca to work toward multiculturalism often looks much like co-optation of various non-white traditions. Most problematic in this area is the controversial practice of adopting Native American ceremonies as part of a group's repertoire, thus contributing to the plundering of native peoples which is well under way in this country. An area in which Neo-Paganism as a whole is weak is in understanding the relationship between predominately white, middle-class, well-educated people seeking personal growth and the complex religious systems of Native Americans, Afro-Caribbean, and South American cultures. Currently, the tendency is for Neo-Pagans to take bits and pieces from these complex systems and to use the pieces for their own personal growth or to attempt to make their environment more healthy. This approach, while well-meaning, ignores the reality of the cultures which are often living in poverty and extreme social stress. Feminist Wiccans need to extend their analysis of class and cultural oppression to the cultures from which Neo-Pagans tend to "borrow" material and to develop a sense of respect for the boundaries set by religious leaders of these other cultures. Native American leaders across the country have spoken strongly against the co-optation of Native ceremonies, especially as taught by people who claim to have been instructed by "wise old medicine people." Weekend workshops which teach people to lead sweatlodges or to invoke Native deities are seen as exploitative by these Native leaders. In the words of one Cherokee woman, "You took our land, you took our children, you took our language, you took our culture, and now you want God?" (C. Kasee, personal communication, September 15, 1991). However, most feminist traditions explicitly try to reduce homophobia, ageism, and ableism within their writing and practice, and are aware of the difficulties experienced by survivors of rape and incest, and by recovering drug or alcohol abusers. Published rituals often make explicit ways in which to build in accommodation for a wide range of circumstances or abilities in ritual participants.

Meeting other Pagans or Wiccans can sometimes be difficult, as neither form of spirituality includes proselytizing. Most Pagans and Wiccans believe that those who are meant for the path will find people to teach them. Responding to or placing ads in local pagan newsletters is one way to make contact; in larger metropolitan areas there are often public rituals or classes advertised. Sometimes women's bookstores will have notices posted about the formation of women's spirituality groups or classes. In any case, while most contacts are well-meaning, discretion is advised when making new contacts.

Identifying as Wiccan involves a process of identity development and management which is in some ways analogous to the "coming out" process that gay men and lesbians experience (Cass, 1979). While some people choose to pursue Wiccan spirituality after exposure to books, classes, or friends, others experience a sense of "coming home," of finally encountering a system of spirituality which speaks to their deepest spiritual needs. Often, after some initial exposure to Wiccan material, people seek out written material, other people, classes, or groups to continue the process of identifying as a member of a non-dominant religious group. Encounters with others may be positive or negative; if no suitable local community is available, people may develop a sense of community through subscribing to the many newsletters, journals, and magazines available, through collecting Pagan music and art, and when possible, attending regional festivals.

As people begin to commit more strongly to a Pagan perspective, their values and sense of who they are begins to change. Most people report an increased sense of responsibility for ecological issues, and many experience a sense of uncertainty as they move beyond the Christian norm in our culture. Wiccan holidays are different than Jewish or Christian ones, which often results in the need to decide whether to miss festival days by going to work or school, or to "come out" to one's workplace in order to keep festivals. Family members may not understand or approve of their loved one's new orientation; some people cope with this by keeping their identity secret, and some disclose and face the consequences. There have been incidences of people losing their jobs, having their homes threatened, and losing custody battles over the issue of their identity as Wiccan, because of the confusion about whether Wicca is a form of Satanism. Because Satanists use some Wiccan traditions, such as the pentacle, night meetings which involve robes, candles, drumming and chants, and because Satanists hold rituals on some of the same holidays, people are sometimes alarmed by what they hear about Wiccan practice. Wiccans work on an individual and organized basis to educate the public about the fact that Wicca is a life-affirming nature religion which has nothing to do with Satan, as Satan is a Judeo-Christian concept. Recently, Wiccans in prison and in the military have been granted permission to practice while within their institutions, although those rights are not always enforced. Like lesbians and gay men, who may seek high visibility at some point in their identity development, Neo-Pagans in the process of identifying as such often wear symbols or clothing that advertises their perspective, may "come out of the broom closet" at work, and may become politically active. This is similar to Cass's model of homosexual identity formation; at this stage, all Pagans are seen to be preferable to all non-Pagans, and there is some tendency at this time to work through the full implications of rejecting a Jewish or Christian identity in our culture. Eventually, the worldview, practices, and identity that develop as a person works through the process of identity formation become integrated into the person's identity as a whole. While being Wiccan is no longer the most salient aspect of the person's identity, it is also not an aspect that can easily be rejected or denied.

While Wicca is a hobby or interest for some people, who look into it and then move on with little change in their lives, for many people becoming Wiccan involves significant change in the way they understand the nature of their world. The Judeo-Christian perspectives which are prevalent in our culture hold that time is linear, that people live one life on earth, that the earth is a "vale of tears" and a place to be endured, used, and exploited, and that women are of little value. While there have been sects of Judaism and of Christianity which have worshipped female aspects of God, including the Shekinah and Sophia, the prevalent view in American culture does not allow for any feminine form of deity. Wiccan perspectives generally believe that time is cyclical, that people live many lives, that the earth is sacred, and that all people are to be honored, male and female, gay and straight, old and young.

Feminist Wicca has the potential to empower women in a variety of ways, through providing positive images of powerful women in the Wiccan community, through teaching women the full range of their potential through understanding aspects of the Goddess, and by providing a community with opportunities to learn different skills and to build strong, sustaining relationships. As an alternative value system to the Judeo-Christian perspective with which most of us are raised, it provides respect for women and for the earth and rejects the notion that humans have the right, privilege and responsibility to dominate and exploit the resources of the earth and its creatures. It encourages people to work to empower themselves and each other rather than to strive for "power-over" others (Starhawk, 1987). It encourages individuals to take responsibility for the effects of one's actions, and to act for the good of the whole, without manipulation or exploitation. Its focus on the agricultural cycle of festivals encourages appreciation of and care for the environment, and its celebration of diverse lifestyles and identities allows the community to draw on the resources of many different kinds of people. As therapists and psychologists who study what is important in women's lives, an understanding of feminist Wicca can provide resources for the empowerment of women clients, as well as men, and can encourage societal change toward the kind of valuing of the environment that we will need in order to survive.

NOTE

Women who are interested in learning more about the Wiccan community and feminist spirituality can make contact through books, through subscribing to newsletters, through attending festivals, or through meeting others who are actively practicing. The bibliography lists several books which are useful at the introductory level; these include Starhawk's *The Spiral Dance,* Z. Budapest's *Holy Book of Women's Mysteries,* Diane Stein's *Women's Spirituality Book* and *Stroking the Python, Ariadne's Thread: A Workbook of Goddess Magic* by Shekinah Mountainwater, and for an overview of the variety of Neo-Pagan practices in this country, Margot Adler's *Drawing Down the Moon.* All of these books include additional resources from which women can draw in order to learn more; several of these writers have written other books, and there are many good sources of information available. A major Wiccan/Pagan newspaper is *Circle Network News,* also listed in the bibliography, which includes articles, networking, classifieds, and information about the larger pagan community. *Tides,* from the Boston area, and *The Beltane Papers: A Journal of Women's Mysteries*, are also high-quality publications. Most publications can be sampled for a nominal fee, and the larger publications usually carry information about smaller, local publications in which women can find local groups and activities. Festivals abound year-round, although particularly in the summer. The largest summer gathering is probably the Pagan Spirit Gathering, a week-long festival held in Wisconsin; there are also week-long camps and frequent training opportunities by various well-known Wiccan leaders.

REFERENCES

Adler, Margot (1986). *Drawing down the moon*. Boston: Beacon Press.

Beltane Papers: A Journal of women's mysteries. 1333 Lincoln St. #240, Bellingham, WA 98226.

Bolen, Jean S. (1984). *Goddesses in every woman: A new psychology of women*. San Francisco: Harper & Row.

Budapest, Zsuzanna. (1989). *The holy book of women's mysteries*. Berkeley: Wingbow Press.

Cass, Vivienne. (1979). Homosexual identity formation: A theoretical model. *Journal of Homosexuality, 4* (3), 219-235.

Circle Network News. Circle, P. O. Box 219, Mt. Horeb, WI 53572.

Dienhart, A. & Avis, J. (1991). Men in therapy: Exploring feminist-informed alternatives. In M. Bograd, (Ed.), *Feminist approaches for men in family therapy*. New York: Harrington Park Press.

Estes, Clarissa P. (1992). *Women who run with the wolves*. New York: Ballantine.

Ganley, Anne.L. (1988). Feminist therapy with male clients. In M. Dutton-Douglas & L. Walker, (Eds.), *Feminist psychotherapies: Integration of therapeutic and feminist systems*. Norwood, NJ: Ablex.

Guiley, Rosemary. (1989). *The encyclopedia of witches and witchcraft*. New York: Facts on File.

Kasee, Cindy. (1992). Personal communication.

Mountainwater, Shekinah. (1991). *Ariadne's thread: A workbook of Goddess magic*. Freedom, CA: The Crossing Press.

Rich, Adrienne. (1980). Compulsory heterosexuality. *Signs, 5* (4), 631-660.

Starhawk. (1979). *The spiral dance*. San Francisco: Harper & Row.

Starhawk. (1987). *Truth or dare*. New York: Harper & Row.

Stein, Diane. (1986). *The women's spirituality book*. St. Paul: Llewellyn.

Stein, Diane. (1988). *Stroking the python*. St. Paul: Llewellyn.

Surrey, Janet L. (1991). The "self-in-relation": A theory of women's development. In J.V. Jordan, A.G. Kaplan, J.B. Miller, I.P. Stiver, & J.L. Surrey, (Eds.), *Women's growth in connection: Writings from the Stone Center*. New York: Guilford.

Tides, P. O. Box 1445, Littleton, Massachusetts 01460-9998.

SECTION III:
LIVING IT OUT

Women's Spirituality and Healing in Germany

Marianne Krüll

SUMMARY. The author first describes her personal experience of celebrating the eight holy-days of the year's circle together with a group of women over a period of several years. The healing power of ritual ceremonies in the spirit of the Goddess is shown through examples of the psychodynamics of the group and of individual women. Differences between consciousness-raising and therapeutic groups are discussed. In a brief review the women's spirituality movement in Germany is presented, mentioning some of the leading healers and writers. In conclusion a comparison between the German and American female spirituality movement is attempted.

This is our ninth year that we, a group of women living in Bonn, Cologne, and Dusseldorf, are coming together to celebrate the year's

Dr. Marianne Krüll teaches a sociology seminar at the University of Bonn. Mailing address: Graurheindorfer Strasse 16, D-53111 Bonn, Germany.

[Haworth co-indexing entry note]: "Women's Spirituality and Healing in Germany." Krüll, Marianne. Co-published simultaneously in *Women & Therapy* (The Haworth Press, Inc.) Vol. 16, No. 2/3, 1995, pp. 135-147; and: *Women's Spirituality, Women's Lives* (ed: Judith Ochshorn, and Ellen Cole) The Haworth Press, Inc., 1995, pp. 135-147; and: *Women's Spirituality, Women's Lives* (ed: Judith Ochshorn, and Ellen Cole) Harrington Park Press, an imprint of The Haworth Press, Inc., 1995, pp. 135-147. Multiple copies of this article/chapter may be purchased from The Haworth Document Delivery Center [1-800-3-HAWORTH; 9:00 a.m. - 5:00 p.m. (EST)].

135

circle, that is, the eight holy-days of the year which our non-Christian ancestors also used to celebrate: (1) the 2nd of February, Feast of Light (Candle Mass); (2) the 21st of March, Spring Equinox (Easter); (3) the 30th of April, Beltane (Walpurgis); (4) the 21st of June, Summer Solstice; (5) between the 5th and the 15th of August, Feast of Cutting and Consecration of Herbs (Harvesting); (6) the 21st of September, Fall Equinox (End of Harvesting); (7) the 1st of November, Halloween (Feast of Darkness); (8) the 21st of December, Winter Solstice (12 or 13 Holy Nights).

In the beginning our group was larger, but even now we are still nine women circling around. In age we now range from 33 to 57. Most of us are married, mothers of one to five children. In one year we had three babies in the group celebrating with us because the mothers were breast-feeding them! Others are beyond the mothering age, living alone.

When we started most of us did not know the others. All of us had the wish to learn about "the Goddess" as she was celebrated and honored in pre-patriarchal times or societies. From various sources we had heard about women's spirituality and wanted to experience and live what we had read or heard. Starhawk's *Spiral Dance* (1979) had been the main source for most of us. (We still chant from Starhawk in English: "We all come from the Goddess and to Her we shall return. . . . ").

Some of us are of the Protestant faith, others Catholic, one is a Buddhist, several have left their former religious affiliation. Some of us are academic women (theologians, sociologists, teachers) who began to integrate women's studies into our fields, discovering our lost heritage. Others in our group are artists: a silk-painter, a performance actor, a meditative dance teacher. One is an expert in herbs and mushrooms. One knows much about astrology. One of us works in an educational institution and thus is in a position to invite prominent women for lectures and seminars. So, we have worked with Zsuzsanna Budapest and Felicitas Goodman from the United States, as well as with Luisa Francia, Gerlinde Schilcher (Judith Jannberg), Ute Schiran, and others from Germany. Thus, the expertise of each of us is shared by the others.

But more important than our sharing of knowledge has been our group process over the years. Mostly our meetings last one day;

some last two or three days. We prefer to be outside, sleeping in tents or under the sky, but in winter we mostly celebrate in homes, some rented, some our own apartments or houses.

We usually start with a power-circle to protect us and raise our energies: holding hands and in silence calling the Goddess to be with us. Then follows a "go-round" to allow each of us to report what has happened to her since we last met. The others ask questions but refrain from interpreting or commenting. Sharing our pains and joys in our everyday lives has, in itself, a profound supporting and healing effect.

Usually a go-round lasts for several hours, so that afterwards we all need some food before continuing. Although we never plan what kind of food each one should bring, there is always just the right combination of dishes for a lavish meal or several meals when we meet for more than a day. We all take pride in preparing new dishes to surprise the others. The food is also a way for us to materially and symbolically connect with the current season of the year.

The ritual we celebrate depends on the respective holy-day and on what one or several of us particularly need, as expressed in the go-round. It may consist of our just gathering in a circle with our symbols for the four corners of the sky and the four elements in the center: a candle to represent the South and the element of fire; a bowl of water for the West; a stone for the North and for the element of earth; a feather or knife to represent the East and the element of air. But a ritual may just as well consist of several parts, such as performances, trances, dances, chanting, drumming, massaging, tarot-reading, or–particularly if we meet for more than a day–the production of objects (like woodcarvings, painted silk scarves, clay figures). Working with our inner images may alternate with the outward staging of some kind of performance.

Sometimes one or several of us are in charge of the ritual, having planned it in advance. More often we create the ritual spontaneously. Here are some examples:

1. Candle-mass in February is the time of the beginning light, of clarity and vision. As a ritual we make our candles for the next year. Bee's wax is heated and while we "draw" our candles by dipping the wick into the liquid wax, we express our

wishes for the next year. The candle keeps our "light" burning in times of darkness throughout the year. One candle is made for the whole group. The color for this feast is white.

2. Spring Equinox is a happy holy-day when tender green sprouts start to peep out of the ground and the first spring flowers are in blossom. We prepare the ground to put seeds in it, and ask Ostara, the Easter-Goddess, to let them grow. It is a time for cleansing, so one year we took baths and dried each other in a soft massage. The color is yellow.

3. Walpurgis is the feast to celebrate the new life in orgiastic joy. It is said that the witches used their broomsticks to fly to the "Blocksberg," a mountain in central Germany. We always try to be in the open, making a fire and jumping over it, dancing, chanting, and feeling the power of spring in us and around us. It is a feast of all colors.

4. Summer Solstice is the year's "high-time" (in German: Hoch-Zeit, also meaning "wedding") when the Goddess and her hero join their power in erotic ecstasy. Mostly, we spend several days together celebrating the abundance of life. The color is a bright red.

5. Cutting the grain and the grass is the theme of the cutters' holy-day. We pick herbs to be dried and kept in our homes throughout the year for protection. One year we killed a hen in a ritual to experience our power as "cutting" women, as women giving death. To some of us this meant a new form of healing: cutting off what needs to be killed in order to feed us or make room for new life. The color is a dark red.

6. Fall Equinox is harvest-time. We give thanks to the Goddess for the goods She has provided us. In one year we had three newborn babies in our midst to be grateful for. It is also a time to give back to mother earth what she needs, particularly in our times of violation and abuse of her resources. The color is brown.

7. Halloween for us is the beginning of the dark season when we honor and meet our ancestors (All-Saints' Day in the Catholic Church), but when we also encounter the shadow in ourselves. One year we spent some hours in a grave-yard in the dark,

each having to deal with her fear of the place and of her own death. The color for this feast is black.

8. Winter Solstice is the longest night, but also the birth of light. It is a time when the skies are open for good or bad spirits to reach out for us. We perform our ritual to get in contact with the spirits surrounding us. Once we spent the whole night outside wearing masks and dancing around a big fire making noise to chase the evil spirits away. In the morning we climbed up a hill to greet the rising sun (which, however, stayed hidden behind clouds!). In another year we celebrated Winter Solstice inside with a birthing-ritual during which every one of us found her way through the tunnel which the others had formed with their bodies. For one of us this was a special form of healing since she had just had a hysterectomy. We guided her through her despair of no longer being able to give birth–as helpful and compassionate midwives would help a child to a new life. Colors are red, green, and gold.

In closing our meeting each of us draws a tarot-card from Vicki Noble's (1983) *Motherpeace* tarot-deck which we spread out in a circle. The card gives us an orientation for the time until our next meeting.

It is difficult to explain what kind of healing we have been getting from our ritual celebrations throughout the years, because most effects are indirect or too subtle for clear observation. I shall try to name some that have been most obvious to all of us.

We have learned to open our senses to the cyclic nature of our lives and of nature around us. This has affected our physical cycles. Menstruating women, for instance, bled at the same time, for some periods even at full moon. Birth-giving was a beautiful experience for the women who had babies (altogether nine women during the past eight years!), some of whom gave birth in their homes.

All of us went through personal crises which were eased and even solved through the help of our group. There were separations from partners, unhappy love-affairs, deaths of close family members. There were illnesses and depressive states with suicidal tendencies. There were breakdowns due to crises at work. We helped each other, through just being there and feeling deeply connected with the woman in sorrow.

Rosemarie (names have been changed to protect confidentiality) had been sexually abused as a child by her psychotic grandfather. She did not remember this and was unable to relate her adult problems to that experience. During several meetings we stood by her when her traumatic experience started to rise to her consciousness and she screamed in terror. She is strong and powerful now, with no signs of depression, mastering her quite difficult life admirably.

When Hilde got pregnant from a casual love-affair she was desperate because an abortion seemed impossible for her, although a child would have ruined her life plans. We held her and cried with her, but also talked to her. When she decided to have the abortion, one of us accompanied her to the doctor's office and to the hospital. At our next meeting we celebrated a mourning ritual asking the child's soul to forgive her and transform her sorrow into power. She is now studying and has taken charge of her life.

Monika is a single mother. She gave birth to her daughter at the home of Sabine. Some women of our group were present, and also Sabine's two children. Monika's daughter is now like a sister to them. Monika is convinced that her beautiful relationship with her daughter (now almost 5 years old) would never have been possible without our group.

There were also controversies in the group. For quite some time Carla and Katharina struggled about who had more to say in the group. Again the group offered support and security for both of them to open up and admit that deep down they had been longing for the understanding of the other instead of fighting her. The power-structure of the group changed enormously after that clarification.

Another constant problem has been to find safe places outdoors for us to meet, since in the overpopulated area where we live there is practically no place in the woods, the fields, on hills or in valleys, in caves or in castle ruins, where we can be sure of nobody coming by. Sometimes we have even been chased away from places we found.

We also had to say good-bye to several women in the group. They left for various reasons, some painful for the rest of us. We keep in contact with them, and the door is open for them to return. It was important for us to learn that separation can be overcome without bad feelings.

What is the difference between our group and other consciousness-raising or therapeutic women's groups? I think it is our spiritual orientation. We do not only come together to help each other, but for some "higher" or "other" purpose which is not easily explainable. We call it "the Goddess." Everyone of us feels that the spirit of the Goddess is with her or even that she is the Goddess. We feel connected with nature around us, with stones and rocks, with plants, animals, other human beings, with the whole cosmos. In the spirit of the Goddess, we accept and respect who and how we are, and we respect the other in her way of being. We may not always like how we or the others are, but knowing that the Goddess is with us, we feel that we have responsibility for "constructing" ourselves and our world in a meaningful way.

This spiritual orientation is our mutual bond and probably explains why our group has stayed together for such a long period. We feel that we are not just good friends, but that we are, so to speak, called to join our energies so that they may grow—not only for our own benefit, but for the benefit of a larger whole.

Another difference from therapeutic groups is that there is no leader in our group. Whenever one of us shows some kind of superiority over the others, she is lovingly criticized by the others, and immediately returns into the circle of equals.

It is amazing how "good or bad" and "right or wrong" change their meaning when you no longer try to hold on to *one* truth, as our therapeutic, religious, and scientific patriarchal belief systems force us to do. Having had academic training myself, I feel tremendously relieved to no longer have to force myself to decide which is right and which is wrong, but to be able to let things and living beings be as they are. For the theologians in our group the change is even more profound. Instead of God-Father up above watching us and punishing us for our wrong-doings, we know that we are responsible for our deeds. As the witches say, "Whatever we do will come back threefold to us," so we better be careful not to do what we do not wish to be done to us!

A very important aspect of our spiritual work is a re-definition of

womanhood. Although we continue living in patriarchal structures–
most of us in marriages, having children of both sexes–we do not
define ourselves as mentally or spiritually dependent on men. We
reject men's definition of women as either whore or saint, sexual
object or mama.

The threefold Goddess–maiden/amazon, mother, crone–is our
self-image as women throughout the life-cycle. The maiden-God-
dess in mythology (e.g., Artemis/Diana, Athena) is adventurous,
unattached, a virgin in her spirit, although she may be active sexually. The mother-Goddess (e.g., Demeter, Hera) is nurturing, creative, giving birth to children, but also to products of any kind. The
crone-Goddess (e.g., Hecate) is the wise, the experienced one who
knows the secrets of life and death. Such positive images of
women's strength have profound healing effects.

We feel that our lives are cyclic: the daily cycle with the sun
rising and setting; monthly with the moon waxing and waning and
with our bleeding coming and going; and seasonally through a
year's cycle. But just as those cycles return, some of us believe that
our own life cycle from birth (or even from conception) to death
will return. And those of us who do not believe in reincarnation
trust that we are in contact with our ancestors, particularly the
female ones.

Our bodies are a source of knowledge and understanding for us.
We reject the notion of a separation between body and mind and
experience enormous strength in healing ourselves without medical
help through visualization, rituals, meditation, and trance. Some
years ago I would never have imagined recovering from influenza
or even seeing an open wound heal as quickly as it happens now
with my "magic" power. Dreams are another important source of
knowledge. We share them in the group and often find a deeper
understanding for ourselves, especially when we dream of one
another or of our group.

There is an opening of all of our senses making us aware of our
reality inside and outside of us. We found that fears disappear and
positive energies arise when we become more aware of what we
hear, observe, and feel. For example, walking at night or even
sleeping in the open is no longer a problem for any of us as it had
been before.

We made several trips together as a group in search of power-places and sites of Goddess-worship. We went to the isle of Malta in the Mediterranean Sea to feel the magic of the magnificent megalithic temples which all have the form of women's bodies. We were on the isle of Rugen in former East-Germany, where we danced on grave-mounds and flew with the swan-goddess–the swan being the sacred bird of the ancient people there. Last year we got to know the spirits of the Alps, and found a "witch-rock" high up above a valley. This year we plan a trip to Cornwall, England, with its many magic places.

THE WOMEN'S SPIRITUALITY MOVEMENT
IN GERMANY

The history of the German women's spirituality movement has not been written yet, so my report can only reflect a very personal view of mine. Also, I can only talk about West-Germany, since I am not informed about groups in the former G.D.R., which, I am sure, do exist by now.

The women's spirituality movement had its roots in the political feminist movement following the students' revolt in 1968. In the late 70s some active feminists discovered that in patriarchal systems women are not only oppressed openly (e.g. economically, sexually, politically) but also mentally and spiritually.

Schiran is a family or clan-name chosen by five lesbian women who in the early 1980s decided to leave patriarchal structures and live on farms in the countryside of Southern Germany. Ute Schiran, a spiritual healer and teacher, a lecturer and author, is the best known of them. Together with her clan-sisters she wrote a beautiful astrological book for women (Schiran, 1985). This and other work of the Schiran women (1988, 1990a, 1990b) have had considerable influence in the German feminist spirituality movement.

Heide Göttner-Abendroth is another leading figure in the movement. She was an academic philosopher who quit her university career. Together with a collective of women she founded an academy for matriarchal living and studies in Southern Germany, called "Hagia." In 1983 she started celebrating rituals in large groups. Many women who took part in her ritual gatherings are now working on their own. Göttner-Abendroth is the author of several books (1991, 1988, 1980) which have greatly inspired the German spiritual movement.

Luisa Francia is another well-known German healer. Her first book *Moon, Dance, Magic* (1986) was a revelation to many of us. Luisa is a wild woman, a true witch with enormous power. (Quite recently, in 1992, she survived a motorcycle-accident by using her spiritual, magical power so that the medical doctors admitted that her healing was a miracle.) Luisa lived in Africa to study witchcraft with native women. She is a productive and witty writer and lecturer (see Francia, 1991a, 1991b, 1989).

Judith Jannberg's book *I Am a Witch (Ich bin eine Hexe)* (1983) opened up a door for many of us to identify with our medieval sisters, the wise women, who had been persecuted and killed as witches. We learned to be proud to call ourselves "Hexe" (witch), meaning "hagazussa," the one who is riding on the fence between the worlds.

There are many centers in Germany where spiritual women healers are working. The "Arkuna-Frauenzentrum" is a fairly new (since 1988) women's project near Stuttgart offering seminars in various fields with the purpose of enhancing women's power.

Aside from these more prominent women and institutions in spiritual healing, there are a growing number of individual women and groups doing their healing work in their local surroundings. In 1993 some 50 women working professionally in the spiritual field gathered in a women's center near Cologne to exchange ideas and to get to know each others' work. Their field of activities include healing through ritual, tarot and I-Ching reading, astrology, yoga, meditative dancing, self-assertion courses, organization of travels for women, and women's history. A congress will be held in November 1994 to promote networking.

Since the demand for spiritual healing is obviously growing among women, such networking seems essential. It should, however, not interfere with the autonomy and the spontaneous character of many small groups doing ritual work and giving each other spiritual, psychological, and physical help, similar to the kind of groupwork described above.

THE SPIRITUALITY MOVEMENT–COMPARISON BETWEEN GERMANY AND THE USA

German spiritual women have learned from Americans. Quite a few of them are of European, German-Jewish origins (e.g., Zsuzsanna Budapest and Felicitas Goodman). It is as if German or European seeds had to find the more fertile American soil to flourish and then to come back and nourish us here on this side of the Atlantic! Others, like Starhawk and Vicki Noble, also taught us how to resuscitate our European female heritage.

By now we German spiritual women have developed our own knowledge in our own language. It is time now to develop our spirituality from our own roots. Because, after all, we are living here next to paleolithic caves, next to magic woods and mountains where fairies and Goddesses had their homes, we can celebrate on neolithic graves, in celtic sanctuaries, in temples of Roman Goddesses, not to mention the many female saints in our Catholic churches. Here are the roots of sagas, fairy tales. We can do our research in local historical archives to find out about regional magic beliefs or rituals. We can find places of power in our immediate vicinity.

But of course, we are also haunted by our historical past of millions of witches killed in the fires of stakes. So, in search of our historical roots, we have to confront ourselves with the pain and sufferings of our sisters whose knowledge as midwives and as women of knowledge was destroyed with their lives. In America women have been persecuted, too. But I think it makes a difference if evidence of witch-burnings is present everywhere. On my way to my office I pass by the place in front of the main church where they used to erect the stake to burn women accused of witchcraft. So, I cannot help remembering my sisters every day!

For we German spiritual women there is another equally painful past which is perhaps even more difficult to overcome: our heritage of Hitler's Nazi-Reich. Nazi ideology abused Nordic and Germanic spirituality in order to enhance the "Germanic race." The Nazis celebrated solstices and equinoxes like we do now, they held meetings at holy places, revived sagas of Germanic Gods and Goddesses. So, in order not to be misunderstood, we need to explain and clarify that reclaiming our Germanic roots does *not* mean embracing neo-Nazi ideology!

We must stop being afraid of our power as women. "Macht" (power) is a quality which some German feminists hesitate to claim for themselves. I have the impression that American women are more at ease with taking power and putting it into action. This may be the result of our history where power-abuse had been so extreme.

Reclaiming our heritage as women is, in this sense, not only of therapeutic value for individuals and groups, but for an entire social group it becomes political action. We have to overcome patriarchy in all of its forms: Roman, Christian, Nazi, or its more recent form of industrial capitalism. We have to discover our female strength and healing power not in *his*-toric, but in *her*-storic times! This is a worthwhile and challenging task for all of us, as Ute Schiran (1990) says so aptly:

> I see an ever growing number of women seeking to remember their own powers. I see their courage and radicality in their demand that this earth be treated respectfully and how they themselves lead a life of respect for earth. It is a movement which is growing in spirals and networks–and which will definitely be influential in our hopelessly disturbed world. (p. 24)

REFERENCES

Francia, Luisa (1991a). *Die schmutzige frau (Dirty woman)*. Munich: Frauenoffensive.

Francia, Luisa (1991a). *Die 13. tür (The 13th door)*. Munich: Frauenoffensive.

Francia, Luisa (1989). *Zaubergarn (Magic yarn)*. Munich: Frauenoffensive.

Francia, Luisa (1986). *Mond, tanz, magie (Moon, dance, magic)*. Munich: Frauenoffensive.

Göttner-Abendroth, Heide (1991). *Das matriarchat II, 1: Stammesgesellschaften in Ostasien, Ozeanien, Amerika (Matriarchy, tribal societies in East-Asia, Oceania, America)*. Stuttgart: Kohlhammer.

Göttner-Abendroth, Heide (1988). *Das matriarchat I: Geschichte seiner erforschung. (Matriarchy, history of research)*. Stuttgart: Kohlhammer.

Göttner-Abendroth, Heide (1980). *Die Göttin und ihr heros (The Goddess and her hero)*. Munich: Frauenoffensive.

Jannberg, Judith (1983). *Ich bin eine hexe (I am a witch)*. Bonn: Edition Die Maus.

Noble, Vicki (1983). *Motherpeace: A way to the Goddess through myth, art, and tarot.* New York: Harper & Row.

Schiran, Ute Manan (1990a). Die geschichte der "spirituellen frauenbewegung" (The history of the "women's spirituality movement"). In Irene Dalichow (Ed.), *Zuruck zur weiblichen weisheit*, pp. 15-24. Freiburg: Hermann Bauer.

Schiran, Ute Manan (1990b). *Die wege der wölfin (The paths of the she-wolf).* Munchen (Knaur).

Schiran, Ute Manan (1988). *Menschenfrauen fliegen wieder (Women are flying again).* Munich: Knaur.

Schiran, Ute Manan (1985). *Mutterrecht der sterne (Mother-right of the stars).* Wiesbaden: Inanah-Verlag.

Starhawk (1979). *The spiral dance: A rebirth of the ancient religion of the great Goddess.* San Francisco: Harper & Row.

A Search for Spirituality:
A Mother and Daughter Story

Gloria M. Enguidanos
Gloria E. Law

SUMMARY. A mixture of African, European, and Native Puerto Rican (Tahino) religions form a historical foundation for the beliefs to which Puerto Ricans adhere. This article follows the search for spirituality of a mother and daughter. Although both born in Puerto Rico, mother was raised in the rural mountains of Puerto Rico and daughter was raised among the majority culture of the United States. Their search follows different paths, but the influence of their country is apparent in the rituals they perform and in the integration of their internal processes.

More and more women turn to female spirituality and to rituals that honor the power with which all women are born. These rituals honor the earth as mother, the natural cycles women experience instinctively, and reliance upon their own inner voice as guidance. The building of faith and the reclamation of inner strength helps to peel away the layers, to face the truth of the past and present, and gives courage to heal and transform the pain.

Many Puerto Ricans seem to profess that there is an invisible world surrounding the visible one (Enguidanos, 1993). A mixture

Gloria M. Enguidanos, PhD, is a Psychologist and Professor in Women's Studies at California State University in Hayward, CA. Gloria E. Law is an International Scholar Adviser at the University of California at Berkeley.

[Haworth co-indexing entry note]: "A Search for Spirituality: A Mother and Daughter Story." Enguidanos, Gloria M., and Gloria E. Law. Co-published simultaneously in *Women & Therapy* (The Haworth Press, Inc.) Vol. 16, No. 2/3, 1995, pp. 149-159; and: *Women's Spirituality, Women's Lives* (ed: Judith Ochshorn, and Ellen Cole) The Haworth Press, Inc., 1995, pp. 149-159; and: *Women's Spirituality, Women's Lives* (ed: Judith Ochshorn, and Ellen Cole) Harrington Park Press, an imprint of The Haworth Press, Inc., 1995, pp. 149-159. Multiple copies of this article/chapter may be purchased from The Haworth Document Delivery Center [1-800-3-HAWORTH; 9:00 a.m. - 5:00 p.m. (EST)].

149

of African, European, and native Puerto Rican religions form this historical foundation. A reverence for both the spirit and the soul engenders a sense of fate, a belief that what happens in a person's life is part of that individual's fate which is determined from birth.

The women of Puerto Rico are called Puertorriquenas, Borinquenas, or Boricuas (Boluchen in the native tongue). Little is known about the early women of the island because historians have paid little attention to this area of research. It is important to have an awareness of the history of Puerto Rican women if we are to understand the development of the character that distinguishes us from other Latina groups.

According to Acosta-Belen (1979), the women of the pre-Columbian indigenous society in Borinquen had access to the highest leadership and political posts, that of chieftain by either maternal, paternal, or marriage lineages. The women were taught to handle weapons and to fight in battles during wars. They were able to participate fully in religious ceremonies and rituals. The two main gods the Tainos worshipped were one male, Yocahu, god of heaven who was personified by fire and the sun, and Guabancex, the earth goddess, who was worshipped for her power over crops and the land. Taino settlements were preyed upon by marauding cannibals from other Carribean islands. These cannibals killed almost all the Taino men and raped and kidnapped the women. The year 1493 marked not only the so-called "discovery" of Puerto Rico by the Spanish explorer Colon, but also the beginning of the final atrocities committed against the Tainas. The remaining women were forced into hard labor such as their culture had never known and were also enslaved as sex objects for the pleasure of the conquerors. Because of death and the birth of mixed children the Tainos eventually disappeared as a group. The heritage they left behind was the spirit of independence, strength of character and survivability that has continued to appear in the women of Puerto Rico for centuries. They also left behind a belief that goddesses protect the land from the ravages of tropical storms and invaders.

Another group that influenced the character of the women of Puerto Rico were the black slaves brought in by slave ships when the Taino people began to dwindle. When both Blacks and Taino women who had borne the children of white men were abandoned to raise the offspring alone, they became the first group of women head of households in Puerto Rico. Beliefs in the spirits and goddesses among Tainos was later replenished by the ancestral worship practiced by Puerto Ricans of African descent. Santeria, Espritismo and Espiritualismo are distinct religious forms within the Puerto Rican community. Espiritism is a form of French Espiritism that combines Roman Catholicism and ritual sorcery from Afro-Cuban Santeria (worship of Saints). Spiritualism is a religion characterized by the ability to speak with the dead.

MOTHER'S STORY

I lived with my parents on our sugar and coffee plantation that covered over a hundred acres of beautiful land in the mountains of Puerto Rico. Being the youngest, I stayed with my parents at home while my brothers and sister attended school during the week in the nearby town of San Sebastian. I remember playing solitary games and remember the freedom I had to roam the land by myself. Tropical fruits, flowers, trees and farm animals were my only friends for the first four to five years of my childhood. I learned many folk stories and practices from the peasants or "jibaros." I learned to be aware of "bad spirits" that roamed the earth and learned rituals to protect myself from them.

My mother was the daughter of Catalanes (Catalonia, Spain), a very Catholic family that was considered high middle class. Her father and uncle came to Puerto Rico as medical doctors who had studied at the Sorbonne in Paris. Her father was also a musician who played the clavichord and composed music. My mother was engaged to be married to a man accepted by her family. However, when she met my father they fell deeply in love and due to his unacceptability to her family as a suitor, they eloped. I'm not sure whether they married in the Catholic Church or had a civil wedding. This event may have been the catalyst for her separation from the Church.

My father was born to a distinguished and powerful Gallego family (from Galicia, Spain). The first of his ancestors to come to the island was a general who was sent to be governor of the island by the King of Spain. His nephew was my grandfather who died very young. His death devastated my father, who at an early age left his mother's home after she remarried an alcoholic and abusive man who drank away much of the family fortune.

My father was a very tall young man and was able to pass for older. He secured employment on a gambling boat that travelled between Puerto Rico and Santo Domingo. It was on these boat trips with these island people that he came to learn about and eventually embrace the practice of Espiritismo.

Even though neither of my parents were devout, they were believers in the existence of God. I can't recall ever going to church with my parents individually or as a family. My mother was a classic example of Puerto Ricans assimilating a variety of religious traditions in order to survive a difficult life. She ritually prayed to certain saints that were identified as being helpers with particular hardships. She used a combination of the Catholic ritual of novenas–repeating a prayer for nine consecutive days–and a meditation practice. My mother was devoted to the Virgin Mary and prayed often to the baby Jesus. This reverence for the Virgin is one I seem to have inherited and serves me as a feminine image of the divine. There were all sorts of ritualistic undercurrents in my mother's version of religious practice. She also prayed with the rosary, lit candles for the dead and used holy water in her rituals, clearly paralleling the magical Caribbean religions. She also had a tolerant attitude for those who practiced the rituals of espiritismo like my father whose worship she never tried to stop.

I know very little about my father's ritual worship because he kept the practice secret. I recall some sort of concoctions in jars which he kept high upon shelves near the ceiling. I assume they were kept for protection, although this was never discussed. One practice he had was the use of symbolic crosses formed on our foreheads by his fingers when we were ill. I still recall that touch when I'm feeling ill and need a mental healing image.

Life in my home was very difficult. My father's on-again, off again mental illness hurt the familial sense of well being. Although he was very loving at times, the demons that visited his tortured mind caused him, in turn, to torture his wife and children. It was also difficult for my parents to deal with the issues of raising children within an encroaching modern society. Both my parents were really 19th century people with 19th century values. My parents seemed incapable of understanding the changes in the mores of the new society. As I reached puberty and I started to be aware of my own sexuality, my parents felt as though they were losing control of me and often physically abused me for simply looking at men or even my being noticed by men.

This precipitated my marriage at the tender age of 18 to a man 10 years my senior. He was acceptable to my family because he was Spanish and a professor. I believe now that I was just looking for a way out of the unhappiness and abuse and was not prepared for settling down. I had many dreams of who I could become and I was forced to give them up to become a wife and mother. Approximately four years into the marriage, after the birth of two children, my husband and I immigrated to the United States in order to save our ailing marriage. The relationship continued to deteriorate, but the teachings of my parents, my culture and the Catholic Church said that divorce was evil, and thus I stayed in a union with a man that drank too much and insisted on keeping the family isolated and under his control. We lived in academic communities where I was held up to his colleagues as the supportive wife. I was discouraged from any personal development or friendships. Still, there were good times, such as the birth of our four children, but raising them during the 50s, 60s, and 70s created many of the same ethical conflicts my parents had faced in raising me. As they experimented with drugs and became more and more rebellious, I felt I was losing any vestige of control over our family life. I had immigrated to a country to which I have never felt I belonged, and now it was robbing me of my children and family. Although I am now happily remarried to an Anglo man, my life has been very lonely and I have often felt myself without roots.

In these tumultuous times, rituals have often come to my aid. I still collect water each New Year's Even to capture the bad spirits that may inhabit my house and toss the water out the window at midnight. I continue to light candles to honor the spirit of my dead son and others who have passed on in my life. I have now purchased and am about to move to some land with my husband, finally fulfilling a lifelong dream to return to the earth. I have committed myself to protect this acreage of pine trees and redwoods, planting all native plants to return it as close to its original pristine beauty as possible.

This land and the rituals I practice serve to connect me to the child I was in happier days before the traumas of my life began. My church is the earth and my spiritual enrichment is found in my solitude.

THE DAUGHTER'S STORY

I am a product of multiculturalism and diversity. My mother is Puerto Rican and my father a Spaniard. I myself was born in Puerto Rico and spent most of my life in southern or middle America going to school almost exclusively with people of white anglo saxon backgrounds. I always seemed to stand out and feel different. Since the only other Puerto Rican woman I knew was my mother, I saw my outspokenness and passion–my differences–as idiosyncracies, and sought out people who also felt like outsiders to be my friends.

My home life was a dramatic contrast to that of the people I associated with in the outside world. Most of the people who were my friends were fairly reserved and loved visiting my house because it was intense, vibrant, and full of music, dancing, and good food. There was also the freedom to be open and self-expressing in a way that most of them were denied in their homes. All these things I loved and appreciated about my family and now attribute to our culture. But there was also a dark side to our life at home; alcohol, violence and deep unhappiness. I found myself emotionally drawn to the beauty, intensity and pride of my culture while longing what I perceived of as the normalcy and calm of my friends' home life. All of these experiences fostered in me the deep desire to identify who I was and what I believed in.

I was raised in the Catholic Church. I believe my parents chose this church because they came to that point that many parents do when deciding what they want their children to believe in and need a structure to teach it within. The Catholic Church was the traditional hispanic religion and what I'm sure was the most comfortable option for my parents. It was clear my father was attending church because it was the thing to do as a family. Although he talked of his attraction to the beauty of the ritual, I never thought of him as a believer of the doctrine. Although my mother practiced the Catholic traditions, her obvious independence and fostering of free-thinking encouraged us to question and doubt. I did not understand how the Catholic Church could be the only right church and I railed against the idea that women were relegated to subservient positions. But despite my rebellious nature, I was strongly affected by the concept of a judgmental God and came to believe that if I was just a good enough little girl, my life would improve, family problems would go away, and I would not feel so different and alone.

Although I rarely attend a Catholic church these days, I remember not only my favorite parts of the mass, but also the emotion and awe I felt as I heard the Latin words, smelled the incense and sang the hymns. At the age of 13, I was finally given the choice by my parents of whether or not to attend church any more. Aside from a short revisit to a liberal church in Berkeley, California, I have never returned. It was easy to leave what for me was a guilt-ridden religious experience.

I spent the next few years attending a wide variety of churches. It was a very interesting religious education, but I never found a church I felt comfortable in. There were still no people of my cultural background, and I found myself in strong disagreement with at least part of the doctrines.

It was during my studies at Indiana University that I first had an inkling of what would eventually become my spiritual and religious practice. I took a Native American religion class taught by a member of the Lakota tribe. I was introduced to the belief that the spirit of God existed in all people and all things. There was little judgement in this religion and a profound respect for the earth. The rituals seemed almost familiar, and it felt as if my soul was expanding and breaking free from its constrictions. Unfortunately, in Bloomington, Indiana in 1971, there was no open practice of native earth-based spirituality and so, although I always remembered what I had learned, I put the knowledge away deep inside me.

It was after several years of marriage and the birth of my two sons that I began to reassess my life. I started to look at what kind of model I was for my children. Through therapy and joining a twelve-step program for compulsive overeating, I was finally starting to define what I believed in. It was in this program that I was encouraged to define God in whatever form I wished.

The first image I came up with was a traditional, patriarchal one: a beneficent, long-haired man who cared for me, listened to me and encouraged me to be exactly what I wanted to be. My father had always been very clear about what he wanted for me to become; this caused me much conflict and pain because I was never asked what I wanted for myself. I believe this new image of God was the father I never had: completely present, supportive and loving.

I began to develop a meditation practice and my image of God began to change. The male image in my meditations was now accompanied by a female image that walked hand in hand in equal partnership. I believe that this was my first, tentative step toward accepting a feminine image of God. The fact that this image was accompanied by a male kept the old voices of my early religious indoctrination happy.

In many ways, during my three years in the twelve-step program, it was my church and community. But this was not a community that I could share with my family. My husband and I started looking for a church for our children in the same way my parents had. Because of our cultural differences (my husband is from a white anglo-saxon background) finding a community we were both comfortable in was very difficult.

When we visited the First Unitarian Church of Oakland, we both immediately felt at home. Here was a church which believed in the inherent worth of every human being, and in social justice, which would offer our children an extended family that included interesting people of many cultures and beliefs, and many of this society's ostracized groups such as gays, lesbians, and the physically challenged. Since the Unitarian Church is not doctrinal, we could both believe what we wanted.

It was as a member of the church that I took a class on non-European goddesses. During the first few classes I heard voices which screamed at me and told me that I was going to hell; vestiges, I'm sure, of my Catholicism. Fortunately, I had the courage to tell those voices to take a hike.

After a while, I started to recognize myself in the practices of women all over the world. I had known for a long time that I felt closest to God when I was in nature and close to the earth. I joined the women who took the class with me in a women's earth-based ritual group.

It was at this point that the memories of the most furious demons of my childhood came back to me. It makes sense that at the time I found the deepest friendships, strongest community and support that I had ever known, I would remember the most difficult parts of my life. These were painful memories I had buried in the deep recesses of my mind. Remembering created my biggest crisis of faith. My new visions of the Goddess were still fragile and I reverted back to embracing a judgmental God. If my life had been, and now continued to be, so difficult, I must not be doing things right.

It was during this crisis that my mother began to talk with me about the history and the strength of Puerto Rican women. She talked about how they had endured horrible abuse and the strength and power they had preserved for our culture. She talked about her own abuse and the things that had sustained her, primarily her love of the land and the ritual that brought her peace. I came to see and feel the gifts of survival and transformation. I saw myself in my lineage and felt in my heart and soul the women that had come before me.

I continued to talk with my mother and surround myself with the women in my ritual circle and other women in my community. I resurfaced from this experience with a profound belief in the power of my history, and for the first time in my life, with an ownership of who I am and where I come from.

In my ritual group I am encouraged to fully participate as a Puerto Rican woman. When I bring my cultural background to the rituals I create for the group, they are embraced and celebrated. We all come without pretenses and are encouraged to search out our own cultural backgrounds and experiment with customs of cultures we are only just learning about. It is in the complete ownership of ourselves culturally and in the honoring of the practices of all women that we heal from our wounds caused by racism, sexism, and abuses that have robbed us of our ancient selves. We recreate the community of women from one of individuals in isolation and competition to one of wholeness, power and unity.

Our group has structure. We commit to a certain number of rituals per quarter. We consider ourselves earth-based and honor the cycles of nature. We also perform rituals of passage for our children, house blessings and any other rituals that a member may feel a need for. Everyone commits to creating the rituals and every ritual has time for sharing our lives. We meet each quarter for planning, airing concerns or conflicts and restating or redefining our goals. This is how we stay healthy and deal directly with changes.

This group has taught me strong positive ways to live and I am always taking what I learn and trying to apply it to other parts of my life. I have finally found a home for my cultural and religious expression both in my church and my ritual group.

MOTHER AND DAUGHTER SEARCHING

Both mother and daughter began searching for the same kind of healing but along separate paths. Although we both knew very generally what the other was doing and searching for, we rarely discussed the specifics. We were not even aware of the incredible parallels in our stories.

We both. have inherited creative, artistic talents. We are both opinionated and risk-takers. In both cases we grew up with a vague sense of our parents' spiritual beliefs and thus searched for something of our own. We both gather our families in the sharing of Puerto Rican foods and cultural holidays. Gloria, the mother, likes to garden and work with clay and incorporates regular personal rituals in her life. Gloria, the daughter, has found her artistic talent in jewelry-making, and creating native art forms and creating both personal and group rituals. Both of us have a special bond with the earth that is instinctive and primal.

Although we are on different paths, we have met many of the same challenges and come to many of the same conclusions. Our vision of God or Goddess is actually quite different. We feel more comfortable using different types of descriptive language. But what remains powerfully clear is that both of us are being drawn, as many of the women around us, to spiritual practices that speak to a deep longing inside us. In our discussions we have learned that both of us feel like we are only beginning and that the search will be ongoing with future transformations. This knowledge inspires us and moves us forward, together.

CONCLUSION

Rituals cause us to come in closer contact with the true essence of who we are, what we believe in, and how we are feeling inside. Healing, on the other hand, is the integration of our internal powers. When we go through the process of healing, we feel the pain and all its symptoms. By feeling the pain and combining it with the strength we can feel in our spiritual practices, we can accept our past and begin to shift the pain because the present is about a new found strength and compassion of ourselves. The wonderful thing about ritual and feminization of spirituality is that both men and women can find a kinder, gentler image of the divine by adopting ancient practices that predate current predominant religions.

Healing through the development of new spiritual practices that incorporate harmony with ourselves and with the earth, speak to an ancient, primal ongoing of our souls.

REFERENCES

Acosta-Belen, E. (Ed.) (1979). *The Puerto Rican Woman*, Introduction (pp. 1-7). New York: Praeger Publishers.

Enguidanos-Clark, G.M. (1986). *Acculturation, Stress and Its Contribution to the Development of Depression in the Hispanic Women*. The Wright Institute, Berkeley, California, Unpublished Doctoral Dissertation.

Mother Mary Ann Wright:
African-American Women, Spirituality,
and Social Activism

Patricia Guthrie

SUMMARY. The role of African-American women in community service and social activism is well known. In this paper, the researcher provides a case study of a present-day African-American social activist and makes comparisons with the community service experiences of other African-American women in the past. Mother Mary Ann Wright describes herself as a servant of God. As with other African-American women, it is God who provides her identity and sense of purpose. Likewise, because she serves God, she has status in her community. Mother Wright is an exceptional woman–born in abject poverty, having pulled herself up by her bootstraps–all the while listening to the voice of God, she has founded missions throughout the world and is best known for her work in feeding the hungry in the parks of Oakland, California. She gives all credit for her accomplishments to God. However unique and outstanding, Mother Wright also epitomizes a long tradition of African-American women whose spirituality directed their service to their fellow human beings. The list is long and the variety of these women is great–the well educated leaders as well as the ordinary–Pauli Murray,

---

Patricia Guthrie earned her PhD from the University of Rochester in Social Anthropology. Her forthcoming book *Mother Mary Ann Wright: Angel of the Poor* is based on two years of field research. Currently, she is Director of Women's Studies and Assistant Professor of Human Development at California State University, Hayward.

[Haworth co-indexing entry note]: "Mother Mary Ann Wright: African-American Women, Spirituality, and Social Activism." Guthrie, Patricia. Co-published simultaneously in *Women & Therapy* (The Haworth Press, Inc.) Vol. 16, No. 2/3, 1995, pp. 161-173; and: *Women's Spirituality, Women's Lives* (ed: Judith Ochshorn, and Ellen Cole) The Haworth Press, Inc., 1995, pp. 161-173; and: *Women's Spirituality, Women's Lives* (ed: Judith Ochshorn, and Ellen Cole) Harrington Park Press, an imprint of The Haworth Press, Inc., 1995, pp. 161-173. Multiple copies of this article/chapter may be purchased from The Haworth Document Delivery Center [1-800-3-HAWORTH; 9:00 a.m. - 5:00 p.m. (EST)].

161

Mary McLeod Bethune, Sojourner Truth, Harriet Tubman, and thousands of other African-American women have dedicated their lives to uplifting the race and improving the human condition. The story of Mother Wright, a special and exceptional woman in her own right, nevertheless confirms the continuation of the tradition of spirituality and public service among African-American women.

HISTORICAL PERSPECTIVE

African-American women and the social activism tradition, which often is rooted in spirituality, have been largely ignored by traditional scholarship and feminist critique. It is hoped that this discussion will help to remedy that lack.

"Mother Wright," as she is affectionately known, reared 12 children in abject poverty in rural Louisiana and in Oakland, California. Having survived brutal domestic violence, Mother Wright was a domestic worker and cannery employee. In her later years she went on to create an Oakland-based foundation that provides food and shelter to the poor and homeless. In addition to her foundation work, Mother Wright has established missions around the world and has traveled to Africa, Europe, and Asia. She regularly speaks at local schools and universities and has received hundreds of awards and citations.

Why did Mother Wright become involved with the homeless and the poor? She will tell you quite simply that what she does is based on her personal relationship with God. Mother Wright maintains that she has heard the voice of God. God spoke to her when He commanded her to leave her violent husband, and again when He told her to feed the hungry. It is Mother Wright's spiritual relationship with God that frames and defines her local, national, and international work. It is this spirituality that moves her forward and gives meaning, purpose, and direction to her life.

However unique and outstanding she seems to be on one level, Mother Wright is also representative of other African-American women who successfully and effectively moved from the domestic and private domain into social and public service. Despite bitter race, gender, and class oppression, their strong spirituality has empowered African-American women and enabled them to move forward in the struggle against injustice and inequality.

African-American women, in a very profound sense, have shaped the culture of resistance, the patterns of consciousness and self-expression, and the social organizational framework of the local and national expressions of community. Since slavery times, African-American women have been engaged in all aspects of community organization and service–in education, civil rights, organized labor, business, politics, religion, the professions, and club work (Dodson & Gilkes, 1981; Gilkes, 1985; Naples, 1992; Ladner, 1989).

In a racist and sexist society, African-American women like Harriet Tubman, Sojourner Truth, and Mother Wright heard God's voice and struggled heroically to improve their lot. African-American women of the 20th century have been the sources of community endurance, something within that held the reins, enabling them to dream, to serve, and to resist (Dodson & Gilkes, 1981). Organized for community service, African-American women have often maintained that as colored women who had suffered, they are unable to be blind to the suffering of others (Dodson & Gilkes, 1981).

The enthusiasm with which African-American women have taken on the problems of social change and racial injustice has served to energize the African-American community as a whole through the instrument of the African-American church.

Within the African-American community, Holiness and Pentacostal churches are referred to collectively as the Sanctified church. These new denominations never lost their connectedness to the larger African-American religious experience. In spite of the controversies they engendered within the community, the continuity of the Sanctified church within the overall collective religious experience has been of vital importance. These churches today still maintain the charismatic African-Christian worship tradition and linkages to slave religion. The Sanctified church, whose denominations disagreed vigorously over the proper role of women in the churches, nevertheless attracted large numbers of talented, spirit-filled women who felt called to labor in the gospel ministry (Giddings, 1984).

These women migrated from the rural areas to the cities and carried on the movement and organized revivals. Although African-American churches generally are heavily female, by some estimates 75 percent, the Sanctified church is the most female of these churches, with some congregations having 90 percent female memberships (Giddings, 1984; Gilkes, 1986).

Mother Wright is one among a tradition of African-American women who have stood up to be counted. A precursor of Mother Wright, Mary McLeod Bethune (1875-1955) was one of the most powerful African-American women on the national scene. She made an impact on the institutional life of the African-American community and the national policies of the United States. Her entire life was a testimony of service and demonstrated what African-American women could weave out of their sense of Christian duty and calling. She founded the Daytona Normal and Industrial School for Negro Girls at Daytona Beach, Florida. The school which later became Bethune Cookman College had a profound impact on the entire Daytona community and on the lives of such individuals as the noted African-American theologian Howard Thurman (Dodson & Gilkes, 1981). Like Mother Wright, Mrs. Bethune was a woman of deep faith and that faith was evident in her approach to her role as educator and national leader:

> I leave you love. Our aim must be to create a world of fellowship and justice where no man's color or religion is held against him. Love thy neighbor is a precept which could transform the world . . . I leave you hope. Yesterday our ancestors endured the degradation of slavery yet they retained their dignity. I leave you a thirst of education. We are now making greater use of the privileges inherent in living in a democracy. I leave you faith. Faith is the first factor in a life devoted to service. Faith in God is the greatest power but great faith too is faith in oneself. I leave you racial dignity. I leave you a desire to live harmoniously with your fellow man. I leave you, finally, a responsibility to our young people. (Dodson & Gilkes, 1981, Document 3, pp. 97-98)

Thousands of other African-American women, like Sue Bailey Berman, Holly Murray, Nanny Helen Burroughs, Ida Robinson, Ida B. Wells, Leatine Kelly, Mary E. Jackson, Lucy Campbell, Myrtle Foster, and Mother Wright, have shared something in common–a faith in God and a commitment to service (Dodson & Gilkes, 1981). That commitment to service provides meaning and purpose to their lives and, for these African-American women, is the very basis of mental health.

Mother Wright is a member of the Sanctified church from which she draws her religious faith. It is the church of the oppressed that speaks to the African-American experience. The Church of God in Christ, to which Mother Wright belongs, is the largest of the denominations of the Sanctified church (Gilkes, 1986). Officially a Pentecostal church, it began as a Holiness denomination and has its origins in a dispute among Mississippi Baptists, whose history of independent worship stretched back 30 years before slavery.

African-American women were the most numerous adherents to what Zora Neale Hurston called "a protest against the high-brow tendency in Negro Protestant congregations," the Sanctified church (Hurston, 1981, p. 103). The term Sanctified church provided a cultural and experiential landmark for most African-American Christians (Hurston, 1981). It tends to be a significantly misunderstood segment of a very pluralistic African-Christian religious tradition that we often refer to as "the black church." The Sanctified church carries with it an enormous cultural impact and encompasses those independent denominations and congregations formed by African-American people in the post-Reconstruction South and their direct organizational descendants (Dodson & Gilkes, 1981; Gilkes, 1986; Hurston, 1981).

During the period when African-American people were first making choices about their cultural strategies as freed men and women, the Sanctified church rejected a cultural and organizational model that imitated European and American patriarchy. African-American women built and maintained the churches wherein they have asserted their economic and structural importance. The role of the Sanctified church in the history of African-American spirituality is very important because African-American women carried their Christian missionary zeal beyond the walls of the churches and into the streets, houses, and schools of their communities. For many of these Christian women who wished to be missionaries in Africa, they discovered their own "Africas" right next door (Davis, 1933). The church became a specialized religious institution wherein they organized an array of organizations that addressed concerns ranging from rights of household domestic workers to the problems of international relations and the end of colonialism (Gilkes, 1986).

These Sanctified women organized clubs for youths and homes for unwed mothers. They purchased clubhouses, provided housing for college students, established organizations of cultural refinement for household domestics, organized political clubs, campaigned for women's suffrage, and participated in a wide variety of activities designed to promote social change and to advance the interests of the race (Caulfield, 1974; Davis, 1981; National Council of Negro Women, 1951).

Thus, the story of Mother Wright in Oakland, California, is not an anomaly but rather represents the continuation of an historical African-American women's movement that was motivated by spirituality, directed towards social change, and an instrument for effecting mental health. Highlights of the minutes of the 1941 convocation of the Church of God and Christ provide important insights into the relationship between the women and the church (Document 7, Dodson & Gilkes, 1981).

When Mother Coffey gave her report, there was no mistaking her calling: "I am a servant of the most high God. God gave me this appointment and no man can take it from me" (Dodson & Gilkes, Document 7, 1981, p. 109).

Ladner (1989) described the social responsibility of Black women as a noble tradition of being doers–that is, they were brought up to believe they could do anything. They had to be flexible, to learn to wash, cook, sew, get an education, raise the children, work in their churches and clubs, and anything that needed to be done (Ladner, 1989).

Jet magazine (Booker, 1985) once carried a piece on Mrs. Maime Till Mobley, the mother of Emmett Till. She is also a member of the Church of God in Christ. One of her favorite activities was working with the young people of the church. The author emphasized the importance of Emmett Till's lynching for the heightened consciousness of the African-American community (Booker, 1985).

Grieving and filled with anger at the lynching of her only child, 14-year-old Emmett Till, during a summer trip to Mississippi, Mrs. Mobley defied pressure from local authorities to immediately bury her son. Instead, she demanded that his battered, mutilated body be brought back to Chicago. "Open it! Open the casket up!" she screamed. "Let the people see what they did to my boy!" (Booker, 1985, p. 11). The implications of Mrs. Mobley's insistence that the boy's body be displayed and the attendance of almost a quarter of a million people at the funeral home for a viewing were similar to the consequences of the public funerals in South Africa today. She was able to prevent Mississippi officials from hastily burying the body in Mississippi rather than shipping it to Chicago. Deeply religious, she said, she believed that the Lord knows best. When the Till case was reviewed on Chicago television, she said she felt as though she was encased in a block of ice.

"But then I had a dream," she told a reporter, "I was standing on a bridge as high as any building in Chicago. I looked down at the raging waters far below me, then I heard the Lord say 'I have kept you far above the troubled waters'" (Booker, 1985, p. 12).

Spirituality, religion, and the church are important life features for African-Americans and are important issues in therapeutic as well as social relationships. To highlight the importance of spirituality in mental health, researchers analyzed the relationship between mental health and religion for 114 African-American women. Researchers sought to identify individuals in mental distress and to collect statistically significant and clinically meaningful information for high- and low-religious groups (Handel, Black-Lopez, & Morgan, 1989). They employed an integration scale of the personal religiosity inventory and psychological distress using the Langner Symptoms Survey (an epidemiological measure with a valid cutoff score to identify people in mental distress). A low level of religiosity was associated with significant mental distress, whereas a high level of religiosity was associated with adjustment scores that did not reflect psychological distress. Analysis of data for this sample of women showed both a statistically significant and clinically meaningful relationship between religiosity as measured on the integration scale of the personal religiosity inventory and mental distress for African-American women. For this group, there was a strong association between religion and the presence of psychological distress. Specifically, a low level of religiosity as measured on integration was associated with Langner scores that reflected significant mental distress. High scores on integration were associated with Langner scores, but these scores did not reflect psychological distress.

In the past, white Americans have tended to demean African-Americans as a community of people living outside the law. Undaunted by this form of ridicule, African-American church members referred to themselves as saints (Gilkes, 1985). Without hesitation, the Sanctified perceived themselves to be set apart for sacred purposes. These women and men were confident that God had raised them up for a special calling. Regardless of the intensity of racial oppression, it was the responsibility of the saints to do everything in their power to prevent their oppressors from destroying them (Gilkes, 1985; Tinney, 1981).

FAITH AND MOTIVATION OF MOTHER WRIGHT[1]

By any standards, Mother Mary Ann Wright, the angel of the poor, is an exceptional human being (Guthrie, 1994). She is both unique and inspiring because of the scope of the charitable work she has done. At the same time, she epitomizes a tradition among African-American women who have been motivated to service by their spirituality.

"This morning I had to lift up some heavy boxes. I don't know where I got the strength. I asked the Lord and it was there" (Guthrie, 1994, p. 10).

Why does Mother Wright work so hard for the poor?

"That's easy," she will answer, "the Lord told me to do it. I was lying on the sofa and the Lord came to me in the middle of the night and told me to feed the hungry. I said 'Lord, that's what I been doing, feeding the hungry'" (Guthrie, 1994, p. 12).

Wherever Mother Wright feeds people, there is always prayer, words of hope and encouragement, and spontaneous religious singing. She is often joined by other missionaries and preachers. Mother Wright's life is shaped and motivated entirely by her relationship with God. She listens to God's voice. Because He speaks to her, she

---

1 The following material was collected during two years of taped interviews with Mother Mary Ann Wright.

speaks to others. She will tell anyone who listens just what motivates her and makes her happy.

My great-grandmother was sold by the masters in slavery time. She showed us welts on her back where they whipped her with an eight-ply whip. They put the food in troughs like you pour slop for hogs to eat. They had to eat with they hands down on they knees. She told us that. We ate with our fingers, too. We just used what we had and that was very little, but nobody complained because everybody was on the same level. When you're talking and ministering to people you wonder do they really understand the true meanings of the gospel of Jesus Christ. People are so mean to one another. The Bible say love your enemies and do good to those that spitefully use you. Whatever good seeds you sow, good seeds you will reap, but when you sow bad seeds, you gonna reap bad seeds. He said all souls are mine. He wants us to be like Him. It's a song that said "I wanna be like Jesus, I wanna be like Him" (Guthrie, 1994, p. 106).

I want Him to say [to me], "Well done, my good and faithful servant, you've done great things down here but come up a little higher, I have greater things for you." I can feed all the people in the world and give all the things that people need but unless I live for God, He's gonna say, "Depart from me, I don't even know you," that's what the Lord gonna say if we don't live for Him (Guthrie, 1994, p. 112).

I got married on Christmas day. I never had a wedding ring, not to this day. I married in a purple tunic. When I look back on and remember, it was like yesterday. I was 14. What kind of a life would [anyone] have marrying at the age of 14? No school, no proms to go to, no graduations. Do you know how serious it is to have a baby? I would have my babies and go right back to the fields, we was hoeing, didn't have a change in dress because I didn't have no dress to change in and no shoes on my feet, working with the rag tied on my head. I always had a baby in my belly and in my arms and one hanging on my dresstails. If we would really think about what the good Book say, read the word of God, hear what it say and be a good listener to it and apply to it, a whole lot of things wouldn't be what it is today. One person can't help the world but I tell you one thing, we can put a big dent in it. Put such a big dent in it until others done passed by will remember that you've been there. They'll remember that you've been there. It's just kind of fascinating how God took this little nobody, just a little nobody as I am, a little nothing but the clay and with nothing, the great things that the Lord has done. He has worked His miracles through His little servant (Guthrie, 1994, p. 123).

Oh God, I think about all the troubles and the trials and the tears I've shed. When I think about how far God have brought me, He brought me, He taught me, He saved me, and I'm glad about it today. I cannot let myself forget where the Lord has brought us from. He brought us from the dunghills, from the flat hills of Louisiana, from the cottonfields, when it was so dark we couldn't see nothing. Everything we need, God got it. Everything that you want to do in this life, the Lord provide you with the way to do it. So we of ourselves, we're nothing. People say why don't you get some rest? What do I get in any rest? The Lord has the rest for me. (Guthrie, 1994, p. 125)

How did Mother Wright begin her work to feed the poor? It started with her faith in God. He wouldn't ask her to do something she couldn't do.

I started out kinda begging. I went to the Carnation Company where they had ice cream and milk and I started begging. And then I went down to the produce market at Jack London Square and I'd go from vendor to vendor begging people to give me some food to feed the hungry. Salvation and love you cannot buy, but the Lord allowed me and I said, Lord, it's hard, but thank you for calling me. Out there in the midnight hours we've worked hard together to keep the people warm and we could with what it had taken to sustain them with blankets and sleeping bags. And I was cooking 10, 11 huge pans of food, chicken, string beans, corn, carrots, macaroni and cheese, peach cobbler, candied yams, given them nothing less than the best in their stomachs. And the Lord would keep it steaming hot until I got to the park to serve it. Can't nobody do [for] you like Him. He will fix every condition. Then when you feed these people, they standin in line from three to five hundred and on holidays a thousand or more, when you feed them, you stand back and fold your arms and you say, "Lord, thank you for letting it be me." (Guthrie, 1994, p. 184)

What does it mean to be motivated by faith? What is the relationship between spirituality and mental health?

Many and many a person shared their substance with us. God touches their hearts and *makes them happy.* I used to get upset with the preachers, the Lord Jesus taught more about the poor than He did anything else. How you gonna preach about Jesus and Him being crucified without thinking about how He preached to help the widows and the orphans? This is what Jesus did with the fishes and the loaves. Lord, Lord, when did I see you hungry and didn't give you nothing to eat? When did I see you naked and didn't clothe you? When you did to the least of my little ones, you did it unto me, cause all souls belong to me, He said, all of them, the rich, the poor, the high, the low, all souls. I give honor to the Lord for His many full blessings. I thank Him because He awakened me this morning and kept me with a mind that stayed on Him all day. We love the Lord today because He first loved us. I realize that without Him, we can't do anything.

Without Him I wouldn't be nothing.
Without Him I would fail.
Without Him I would be drifting,
Like a ship, like a ship without a sail.
Without Him I wouldn't be nothing.
Without Him I would fail.
Without Him I would be drifting,
Like a ship without a sail.

When you go out there and all these children, mothers, babies, men, no place to stay, have to sleep in the park under the trees and benches, [knowing] that I am taking a part in their life— *that makes me feel real good,* not pride, not lifting up pride

because you do it, but the spiritual part of love in your heart—
that you were able to reach out to them. We were out there
trying to do what we can to make their lives a little more
pleasant, cause everybody's somebody, there's no big "I"'s
and no little "you"'s—all souls, the Bible say, are mine
(Guthrie, 1994, p. 207).

And now we are blessed with this beautiful shelter, it is like
a show place. We wants nothing less than the best for God's
people. We want to have the brightest light that shines in
America, we just hope that Mr. Clinton will drive by and see
what the Lord has done with His humble servant [Mother
Mary Ann Wright] for the homeless and the hungry (Guthrie,
1994, p. 284).

REFERENCES

Booker, S. (1985, June). Thirty years ago: How Emmett Till's lynching launched
civil rights drive. *Jet*, pp. 11-13.

Caulfield, M. D. (Oct. 1974). Imperialism: The family and cultures of resistance.
Socialist Revolution. 20:2, 67-85.

Davis, A. (1981). *Women, race, and class.* New York: Random House.

Davis, E. L. (1933). *Lifting as they climb: A history of the National Association of
Colored Women.* Washington, D.C.: Moreland Springarn Research Center,
Howard University.

Dodson, J. E., & Gilkes, C. T. (1981). Something within: Social change and
collective endurance in the sacred world of Black Christian women. In R. R.
Reuther & R. S. Keller (Eds.). *Women and religion* (pp. 80-130). San Francisco: Harper & Row, Publishers.

Giddings, P. (1984). *When and where I enter: The impact of Black women on race
and sex in America.* New York: William Morrow.

Gilkes, C. T. (1985). Together and in harness: Women's traditions in the sanctified
church. *Signs: Journal of Women in Culture and Society 10*(4), 678-699.

Gilkes, C. T. (1986). The role of women in sanctified church. *Journal of Religious
Thought 43*, 24-41.

Guthrie, P. (1994). *Mother Mary Ann Wright: Angel of the Poor.* Unpublished
manuscript.

Handel, P. J., Black-Lopez, W., & Moergen, S. (1989). Preliminary investigation
of the relationship between religious and psychological distress in Black
women. *Psychological Reports, 65*, 971-975.

Hurston, Z. N. (1981). *Sanctified church.* Berkeley, CA: The Turtle Press.

Hurston, Z. N. (1978). *Their eyes were watching God.* Urbana: University of
Illinois Press.

Ladner, J. (1989). Black women as do-ers: The social responsibility of Black women, *Sage* 6, 504-506.

National Council of Negro Women. (1951). *Women united: Souvenir yearbook, 16th anniversary.* Washington, D.C.: Moreland Springarn Research Center, Howard University.

Sterling, D. (1985). *We Are Your Sisters: Black Women in the 19th Century.* New York: W. W. Norton.

Tinney, J. S. (1981). The religious experience of black men, in L. E. Geary (Ed.). *The black male.* Beverly Hills: Sage Publications.

A Class That Changes Lives

Robin Powers

SUMMARY. The impact of taking an academic class on Women's Spirituality is examined. The content and structure of the course is described. Numerous examples show that important therapeutic change takes place in the students during the course. From the professor's experience, these changes are greater and different than the ones she sees occurring in a Psychology of Women's class.

For the past twenty-five years there has been a growing interest in an area of study called by various names, depending on one's theoretical orientation, such as feminist theology, feminist spirituality, and women's spirituality. This growth began as women began to enter seminary in greater numbers in the 1960s and early 1970s (concurrent with the growth of feminism and the development of Women's Studies programs) and they became aware that theology reflected only men's experience. When they began to ask about women's experience or wanted to do research about women they

Robin Powers, MA, General Experimental Psychology; PhD, Counseling Psychology, is Assistant Professor, Department of Psychology, West Georgia College, Carrollton, GA 30118.

I wish to thank all of the students who have shared so openly and bravely in my Women's Spirituality classes for the past five years, for this paper could not exist without their help.

[Haworth co-indexing entry note]: "A Class That Changes Lives." Powers, Robin. Co-published simultaneously in *Women & Therapy* (The Haworth Press, Inc.) Vol. 16, No. 2/3, 1995, pp. 175-183; and: *Women's Spirituality, Women's Lives* (ed: Judith Ochshorn, and Ellen Cole) The Haworth Press, Inc., 1995, pp. 175-183; and: *Women's Spirituality, Women's Lives* (ed: Judith Ochshorn, and Ellen Cole) Harrington Park Press, an imprint of The Haworth Press, Inc., 1995, pp. 175-183. Multiple copies of this article/chapter may be purchased from The Haworth Document Delivery Center [1-800-3-HAWORTH; 9:00 a.m. - 5:00 p.m. (EST)].

175

were often ignored or ridiculed (Christ & Plaskow, 1979). But they persevered in their questioning and women (within and outside of the seminary setting) began gathering to discover and discuss their uniquely female experiences concerning religion and spirituality. Experiential workshops occurred and scholarly critiques of patriarchal interpretations of scripture were written (e.g., Daly, 1973; Reuther, 1983). This resurgence (Elizabeth Cady Stanton and The Revising Committee wrote the *Woman's Bible* in 1895 in an attempt to decrease power of biblical authority in the culture because of their perception that scripture was being used to hold women back from equality) in critiquing the Bible goes hand in hand with a rediscovery of goddesses (Stone, 1976), pagan religion (Starhawk, 1979), and cultures that were goddess worshipping and peaceful (Gimbutas, 1991).

The patriarchal world view includes beliefs such as woman as evil, the body as a block to spirituality, and man having dominion over women and children. Its emergence in historic times influences all of us subtly, insidiously, and continuously.

> The lies about the nature and function of woman that are intrinsic to patriarchal religion have informed the legal, educational, political, economic, and medical/psychiatric systems of our society and are accepted as "natural truths" by even the most modern and/or atheistic citizens. (Spretnak, 1982, p. xi)

In contrast to the patriarchal religions, Women's Spirituality emphasizes honoring the body, being aware of the interconnectedness of all things and beings, cherishing diversity, and the embracing of goddess images and attributes and/or a feminist reinterpretation of traditionally patriarchal religions (e.g., Brock, 1988; Daly, 1973; Plaskow, 1989; & Reuther, 1983). In this paradigm man is no longer normative with woman being seen as other (de Beauvoir, 1952). Rather, women are encouraged to explore the depths of their own experience by taking off the filters of the patriarchal paradigm. And, in the past couple of decades, this paradigm with its cherishing of diversity has moved from "woman's" to "women's" spirituality. Within this evolution of consciousness, as more women's voices are heard, a new sensitivity to the racist, ethnocentric, and heterosexist as well as sexist elements of western patriarchal religion is growing.

Because of my scholarly and personal interest in this area I have chosen to teach Women's Spirituality for the past five years in a psychology department (this class is also part of our school's women's studies minor) to a combined undergraduate/graduate level academic class in the rural south. Somewhat to my surprise, I have found that women are profoundly impacted by exposure to this alternative to a patriarchal world view and that this leads to positive changes in their mental health. While I had expected to observe change while utilizing the model of Women's Spirituality in my clinical practice, it had not occurred to me that exposure to this literature in the classroom could change students' lives so greatly.

The goal of this class is to expose students to the literature in the field of Women's Spirituality ranging from the reformation attempts within traditional western religions such as Christianity and Judaism to an exploration of Native American, African and Wiccan spiritual practices. The course includes both didactic and experiential elements. Currently there are many books and/or articles that can be used as texts in classes on Women's Spirituality that may very well lead to the impact upon students described below. For the past several years I have used the following texts in this order: *The Changing of the Gods: Feminism and the End of Traditional Religions* by Goldenberg (1979), *The Politics of Women's Spirituality: Essays on the Rise of Spiritual Power within the Feminist Movement* by Spretnak (1982), *Weaving the Visions: New Patterns in Feminist Spirituality* by Plaskow and Christ (1989), and *Truth or Dare: Encounters with Power, Authority and Mystery* by Starhawk (1987).

This class is usually taught twice a week, each class lasting two hours, for the nine weeks we have available in a quarter. I limit the enrollment to sixteen in order to facilitate discussion and to have time to process imagery work. Since I want this class to be both didactic and experiential, each class starts with the reading of a goddess story (e.g., Stone, 1979) or a feminist interpretation of the Bible (e.g., Fox, 1991; Reuther, 1983), then lecture and discussion, followed by some imagery work. I also use selected videos and

invite a Wiccan High Priestess to be a guest lecturer. The students
are required to write in a journal three times a week responding to
the readings and class, do a take-home midterm, write a term paper
and participate in an oral final (during which we share a meal).

During the nine weeks of this class, unlike any other class I
teach, including the psychology of women, I see changes in self-esteem that amaze me. Women who were ashamed of their body size
suddenly start dressing in bright colors, shy women start talking out
in class, and other women start exploring and sharing their creativity. One woman was so proud of one of her exam answers that she
submitted and had it published in a campus literary magazine. For
the first time, many of them no longer feel "odd" or "weird" for
not fitting into the dominant southern culture. These students are
reading what other women have written concerning what they have
secretly thought or experienced socially, politically, medically, spiritually, and/or psychologically. This validation from the reading
assignments (and the professor) enables them to begin to share with
the class what some of them have kept secret for so long. For others
it is as if a whole new world has become available to them. They
may talk about or discover for the first time their connection with
nature–a topic not readily spoken about in a rural farming community where the use of pesticides is a given and hunting a seeming
birth right. Others talk about their ongoing connection with their
dead ancestors. Others feel free for the first time to share spiritual
experiences that do not fit their fundamentalist upbringing (many of
my students are from the rural south and have had very strict fundamentalist religious training).

And they talk about the harm that has been done to them because
they live in a world informed by western patriarchal religion. One
woman spoke of her father's raping her from the age of four to the
age of 14. When she was 14 a visiting friend found out about his
behavior and told. This young woman's father went to jail for 30
days and then came back home. Shocked, I asked why her mother
allowed him back into the home. Her response was that the church
elders told them they must forgive him or go to hell. While taking
this class she found the courage to write him a letter telling him for
the first time what that experience meant to her. She experienced
this as freeing and felt that telling him her experience allowed her to

go on with her life (up to this point she was consumed by anger that somehow was not resolved by her attendance in an incest survivor's group).

The changes that occur cover many areas. For another woman the sense of interconnectedness of nature and all beings impressed her. She had thought that recycling was silly. At the end of the class she told a story about her nephew throwing a piece of paper on the ground and her telling him he should not do that to mother earth–she had experienced her interconnectedness and it changed her behavior and her perception of others' behavior.

Some students are more private but they share in their journals. One very poignant journal entry was made by a student who was back in our geographic area for the summer. She was majoring in Women's Studies at a university in another state. Much to her dismay, for her religion was important to her, her parents kept telling her she could not be a feminist and a Christian. She spent the quarter struggling to let go of the hell and damnation "tapes" that she had internalized as a child. In her journal she wrote that she had been in therapy for several years trying to deal with her bulimia and had had little success in recovering from this eating disorder. Near the end of the quarter during which she took the Woman's Spirituality class she binged and went to vomit. Much to her surprise she could not do it, for she had begun to love her body and no longer could harm it by self-induced vomiting. Somehow in eight weeks she was able to undo 20 years of conditioning that the flesh is weak and sinful.

Another concept that seems to have a great impact on my students is the contrast between the patriarchal view of menstruation (Leviticus 15:19-30, *The Jerusalem Bible*, 1966) which calls us unclean and Women's Spirituality's emphasis on elemental power. Because of the above mentioned pervasiveness of patriarchal religious thought, these students have never looked at their menstrual cycle as a strength or a gift. It never occurred to them it might have been awe-inspiring to bleed monthly and not die or that women separated themselves at this time because they were so powerful rather than unclean. While they know they can have children, they have had no model of the creatrix to deepen and enliven this process. In contrast, an unmarried student who took this course several years ago is now pregnant with her first child. Unlike many students I have counseled about their unplanned pregnancies, she talks about herself as a creatrix and the child as a gift from Goddess. She too struggles about whether to keep the child or to put it up for adoption but within the context of being a creatrix who does not hate this small being. As we become more sophisticated about psychoneuroimmunology, I can't help but think this attitude of hers has to be good for the health and development of this fetus becoming a baby.

Some of the students choose to reject their religious backgrounds and get involved with various earth religions or develop their own spiritual practices. (Not having longitudinal data I do not know if this is temporary exploration or a more permanent choice.) Being able to hear their own voices and have them validated gives them the courage to hold on to their beliefs in spite of sometimes violent responses from their families. Others find a deeper meaning within their own religious heritage. One woman said that she had always known that Roman Catholicism was the true way and that she still believed that to be accurate. But, for her, studying Women's Spirituality showed that there are many paths to the truth in addition to Roman Catholicism and she felt her world was enriched by this awareness.

Some of the students are or have been in therapy for issues such as eating disorders, incest, rape and so on; others have never been in therapy. But many of them, in both groups, find that when they share their issues as women in this class setting they experience it as very freeing. Their sense of identity becomes broader than that which they, society, and often the self-help/psychological community has been labeling them. For example, they stop calling themselves incest survivors, and begin to see themselves as complex women who have experienced incest. They see that their suffering is due to a patriarchal society that harms all women and men which has adversely influenced their unique family and/or life situations. They learn at a fundamental level that the personal is political.

Many of these students, like most women in our culture, have grown up without female models of strength. When asked to name the hera (or shero) that most influenced them when they were growing up, they are usually at a loss. The most common one named is a personal relative rather than a cultural figure. However, as the quarter progresses and they read about powerful women and goddesses in writings by women, do exercises that get them in touch with their inner female strength, and hear stories about goddesses they begin to discover their power from within and are amazed. Some of them pick a goddess as a model to help them through whatever are their particular issues in this phase of their lives. This combined with the positive emphasis on the female body is empowering. As mentioned above for the first time they look at the natural cycles of their bodies with awe rather than disgust and I hear people telling each other that they are on their moon time rather than that they have the curse. Their body language changes and they walk with dignity and pride. And they, some for the first time, begin to see other women as sisters and allies rather than as competition. Each time I teach this course I witness women claiming their womanhood with pride.

No, not all women who take this class are changed profoundly. But I find it interesting that each time I teach it the waiting list to get into the class gets longer. My colleagues tell me that they have observed a new cohesiveness and closeness among the women students in our department since I have begun teaching this course. This fall a graduate student insisted on a picture being taken of the female faculty and graduate students so she could remember our power as she graduated and moved on in her life.

The initial goal as this volume was developed was " . . . to examine possible therapeutic implications for women engaged in some aspect of feminist spirituality . . . [and] to assess both whether and the extent to which this represents a paradigm shift in conceptions of women's mental health . . . " (NWSAction, Spring, 1993, p. 12-13). I believe that my students would say that Women's Spirituality has had a positive therapeutic impact on them. And from the brief summary of my observations stated above it is clear that I agree. It is important to note that such change can happen in the classroom in addition to the therapeutic setting and/or workshops for several reasons: (1) many women are not in therapy nor would they consider that an option and thus would not be exposed to such ideas; (2) with the upcoming health reforms in this country, therapy may be even less available (especially for minority women and poor women); and (3) the very nature of the class (didactic plus experiential in a group format) seems to have facilitated change for many in a very short period of time. Frankly, I seldom see change happen so deeply and so quickly, even working with the clients I would classify as the worried well.

If taking such a class is as powerful as my observations indicate, our next challenge will be to find a way to get traditional psychology and religion departments as well as more women's studies programs to put it in their curricula. There are few psychology departments like the one in which I teach that intellectually support delving into the transpersonal realms of being, feminist or otherwise.

REFERENCES

Beauvoir, Simone de. (1952). *The second sex.* New York: Knopf.
Brock, Rita N. (1988). *Journeys by heart: A Christology of erotic power.* New York: Crossroad.
Christ, Carol P. & Plaskow, Judith (1979). Preface. In Carol P. Christ & Judith Plaskow (Eds.), *Womanspirit rising: A feminist reader in religion.* San Francisco: Harper & Row.
Daly, Mary (1973). *Beyond god the father: Toward a philosophy of women's liberation.* Boston: Beacon Press.
Fox, Matthew (1991). *Creation spirituality: Liberating gifts for the peoples of the earth.* San Francisco: HarperCollins.
Gimbutas, Marija (1991). *The civilization of the goddess: The world of old Europe.* San Francisco: HarperCollins.
Goldenberg, Naomi R. (1979). *Changing of the gods: Feminism & the end of traditional religions.* Boston: Beacon Press.
NWSAction. (1993). Calls for papers. Spring, 12-13.
Plaskow, Judith (1989). Jewish memory from a feminist perspective. In Judith Plaskow & Carol P. Christ (Eds.), *Weaving the visions: New patterns in feminist spirituality.* San Francisco: Harper & Row.
Plaskow, Judith & Christ, Carol P. (Eds.). (1989). *Weaving the visions: New patterns in feminist spirituality.* San Francisco: Harper & Row.
Reuther, Rosemary R. (1983). *Sexism and god-talk: Toward a feminist theology.* Boston: Beacon Press.
Spretnak, Charlene (1982). Introduction. In Charlene Spretnak (Ed.), *The politics of women's spirituality: Essays on the rise of spiritual power within the feminist movement.* Garden City, NY: Anchor Press/Doubleday.
Stanton, Elizabeth C., & The Revising Committee. (1895). *The original feminist attack on the Bible: The women's bible.* New York: European Publishing Co. (reprint ed. Arno Press, 1974).

Starhawk. (1979). *The spiral dance: A rebirth of the ancient religion of the great goddess.* San Francisco: Harper & Row.

Starhawk. (1987). *Truth or dare: Encounters with power, authority and mystery.* San Francisco: Harper & Row.

Stone, Merlin (1976). *When god was a woman.* New York: Harvest/Harcourt Brace Jovanovich.

Stone, Merlin (1979). *Ancient mirrors of womanhood: A treasury of goddess and heroine lore from around the world.* Boston: Beacon Press.

The Jerusalem Bible. (1966). Garden City, NY: Doubleday & Co.

Women's Empowerment
Through Feminist Rituals

Diann L. Neu

SUMMARY. This article examines the function of ritual in feminist spiritual support groups and describes its therapeutic potential to empower women to make and face transitions. It describes and discusses two ceremonies–reclaiming healing powers after incest and coming out as a lesbian–as examples of individual and collective empowerment.

Many women are creating and joining feminist spiritual support groups to develop their sense of their full selves and to gain strength for social change. This feminist religious revolution aims to empower and heal women, communities and the earth. Groups provide participants a safe place in which to pay attention to sources of spiritual strength and to celebrate rituals such as life cycle transitions and healing.

INTRODUCTION

Sara, a mental health professional in her mid-forties, requests support and assistance in planning a ritual to mark publically her survival of childhood incest.

Diann L. Neu, MDiv, STM, LGSW, is a feminist therapist and ritualist who is Co-founder and Co-director of the Women's Alliance for Theology, Ethics and Ritual (WATER), 8035 13th Street, Silver Spring, MD 20910. She has created and published many feminist rituals that promote women's empowerment.

[Haworth co-indexing entry note]: "Women's Empowerment Through Feminist Rituals." Neu, Diann L. Co-published simultaneously in *Women & Therapy* (The Haworth Press, Inc.) Vol. 16, No. 2/3, 1995, pp. 185-200; and: *Women's Spirituality, Women's Lives* (ed: Judith Ochshorn, and Ellen Cole) The Haworth Press, Inc., 1995, pp. 185-200; and: *Women's Spirituality, Women's Lives* (ed: Judith Ochshorn, and Ellen Cole) Harrington Park Press, an imprint of The Haworth Press, Inc., 1995, pp. 185-200. Multiple copies of this article/chapter may be purchased from The Haworth Document Delivery Center [1-800-3-HAWORTH; 9:00 a.m. - 5:00 p.m. (EST)].

185

Dolores, a single mother in her late thirties, has become pregnant unintentionally. She has decided to make a difficult choice for abortion, and now wants my help in creating a ritual to affirm her decision (Neu, 1992).

Maria, a clergy woman in her late twenties, has said out loud to herself for the first time that she is a lesbian. She has told her friends and family, and wants to plan a ritual to celebrate her coming out and living proudly as a lesbian.

Kathryn, a masseuse and grandmother in her late fifties, has agreed to co-plan the May ritual for her feminist spiritual support group. Since being a daughter and having a mother is a common experience for women and girl children of all classes, races, and nationalities, she focuses the ritual on integrating the daughter/ mother relationship (Neu, 1993a).

Janet, a retired university professor in her late sixties, feels that she is becoming an elder. She wants to invite friends, family and colleagues to a croning ritual that recognizes that she has acquired wisdom in her life (Neu, 1993b).

The needs of these women are similar to those of many others who are creating and joining feminist spiritual support groups to rebalance their sense of themselves, increase awareness of their particular contributions to life, and gain strength for social change. These groups are an emerging phenomenon which provide participants a safe place to pay attention to sources of spiritual strength, to celebrate rituals. These groups enable women to mark life cycle transitions, to heal from violence and to be empowered for personal and social transformation. They connect elements of feminist therapy and feminist spirituality to promote women's well-being.

An important component of both feminist therapy and feminist ritual is assisting women to recognize that they are their own experts, that their lives have meaning, and that "the personal is political." My observation is that women gain therapeutic strength from feminist spiritual support groups, indeed that feminist rituals enhance women's mental health by increasing their balance and strength, energy and comfort.

In this article I will examine the function of ritual in feminist spiritual support groups and describe its therapeutic potential to empower women to make and face transitions. I will look at how feminist therapy and feminist groupwork inform feminist rituals. I will describe and discuss two of the five women's ceremonies I mentioned previously–reclaiming healing powers after incest, and coming out as a lesbian–as examples of individual and collective empowerment.

DEFINING THE ISSUES

Challenged by Sara, Dolores, Maria, Kathryn, Janet, and others like them, and knowing first hand the value of feminist ritual, I began to listen seriously to myself, my friends, my clients, the women in my ritual workshops, and the women in both of my feminist spiritual support groups to learn about women's experiences. I began to understand that some women in their search for wholeness desire to incorporate a spiritual dimension into their therapy and support groups. For these women, both therapy and ritual connect their psychological/social/spiritual selves. For some women, therapy enables them to balance some dimensions of their lives. For others, rituals celebrated in feminist spiritual support groups encourage them to give voice to their own awareness and self-doubt, and to empower and heal themselves.

As I work to name the connections between the fields of therapy and ritual, I question: How do women who participate in the rituals of feminist spiritual support groups experience therapeutic change? When does a woman in therapy benefit from creating a feminist ritual to mark her transition into health and wholeness?

Before describing the rituals of Sara and Maria, a look at feminist therapy, feminist groupwork, and feminist spirituality will illuminate how these principles inform feminist rituals in feminist spiritual support groups, and address women's issues of identity, self-esteem, separation, dependency and empowerment during life-cycle transitions.

FEMINIST THERAPY

Feminist therapy evolved from the emerging feminist consciousness of women in the mental health fields who experienced a growing discrepancy between their own life experiences and what was described by the theories and psychological studies they were required to learn and apply. Properly understood, feminist therapy or counseling is a highly personal and fundamentally political encounter (or series of encounters) between women. It is grounded in woman-woman solidarity and is dedicated to client empowerment.

Feminist therapists differ from non-feminist colleagues in significant ways. Primarily, we espouse change of rather than adjustment to societal standards. We understand that women constitute an oppressed group in our society, and we know the psychological effects on women of oppression from sexism, racism, classism, homophobia, abelism, ageism, and prejudice because of religious or ethnic affiliation. We welcome clients' inquiries about other values, orientations, and methods, encouraging them to become educated and conscientious consumers. We reject stereotypic notions of women and men as limiting, distorting, and unhealthy. We value a relationship of justice with clients, accepting them as partners of equal worth. We understand women have difficulty expressing anger and achieving self-nurturing. We teach the value of female friends. We facilitate and support the empowerment of women; we act as advocates for clients. Sara, Dolores, Maria, Kathryn, Janet and others benefit when mental health professionals operationalize these values. Feminist rituals are influenced by these and other insights from feminist therapy.

FEMINIST GROUPWORK

Feminist groupwork received recognition through the first step in the most recent wave of feminist theory. Consciousness-raising as a method was originally developed by members of feminist groups who helped each other to become fully and critically aware of their situation as women. Their encounters–story-telling and sharing personal stories and life-experiences of joy and suffering with other women–took place in small, unstructured and deliberately non-hierarchial groups with rotating moderators rather than one permanent "leader." This method has spread to innumerable women's groups and caucuses; it has been used effectively on a wide scale throughout the feminist movement. It is basic to feminist ritual groups.

For women, the group is (1) a source of immediate support, where the knowledge that the meeting will take place at all provides them a sense of security; (2) a place to recognize shared experiences and the value to be derived from them; (3) a way of breaking down isolation and loneliness; (4) the source of a different perspective on personal problems; (5) a place to experience power over personal situations with the capacity to change and have an effect on them; and (6) a source of friendship (Butler and Wintram, 1991).

Working together in groups, feminists are reclaiming one of women's particular sources of strength: the commitment to empower others, that is, to participate in interaction in such a way that one simultaneously enhances the power of the other and one's own power. Miller (1991) and Surrey (1991) have renamed this nurturing quality, as it has been traditionally underestimated, trivialized, and misunderstood, and call it mutual empowerment, which connotes the true potency inherent in a growth-promoting, life-enhancing, interactive process. Feminist rituals are influenced by these and other insights from feminist groupwork.

FEMINIST SPIRITUALITY

Feminist spirituality starts with women's own search for meaning and encourages women to reclaim female power. It involves women's actualization of ourselves to be self-transcendent. It teaches women to exorcise our own authority for our own lives in order to say to those in patriarchal authority that they have no power over us. It both recognizes and strives to develop a basic oneness with reality. Women's spiritual quest concerns women's awakening to forces of energy larger than self, to powers of connection with nature and with others to affect the equality of all human beings, and to acceptance of body.

Although different feminists have diverse ideas about feminist spirituality, there are shared themes which shape the feminist spirit. Core characteristics of feminist spirituality include being rooted in women's experiences, placing women at the center, reverencing the earth and all creation, valuing women's body and bodily functions, seeking an interconnectedness with all living things, and placing an emphasis on ritual. Women are orientated to the rhythms of life embedded in both humanity and the planet, to an intuitive and integral connection between the life forces of the earth and its inhabitants. These insights are celebrated in the rituals of feminist spiritual support groups.

FEMINIST SPIRITUAL SUPPORT GROUPS

Feminist spiritual support groups are springing up like wild flowers across the United States and throughout the world. Such groups invite women to share their personal stories, to pay attention to their spiritual journeys and personal well-being, and to raise feminist consciousness of group members for personal and societal transformation. These groups are meaningful while they last, and some, like one I belong to in the Washington DC area, have been in existence for over a decade. Others, just as magically as they begin, end.

Some women are creating and participating in new communities such as women-church, an international, ecumenical movement of local feminist spiritual support groups which engage in ritual and transformation at the personal and societal level (Hunt, 1990; Neu & Hunt, 1993; Ruether, 1985; Schussler Fiorenza, 1983). Others are finding their voices within small feminist circles concerned about spirituality and personal growth, and are challenging religious institutions from within and from without (Winter, Lummis, & Stokes, 1994; Plaskow, 1990). Still others are joining in covens to reclaim matriarchal spiritual sources, such as goddesses and wicca (Starhawk, 1982; Budapest, 1989).

Two recent studies, *Defecting in Place: Women Claiming Responsibility for Their Own Spiritual Lives* (Winter, Lummis & Stokes, 1994) and *Women-Church Sourcebook* (Neu & Hunt, 1993) show that women's spiritual support groups as a movement have a lengthy history and are currently re-emerging in city centers and country corners across the United States and throughout the world. They are empowering women to find our own voices and to speak from our spiritual centers. They are setting in motion a real alternative to patriarchal religions. They are bringing about a paradigm shift in conceptions about what women need to be mentally healthy.

Group connection and ritual, personal well-being and personal transformation, social justice and social identity are some reasons women have stated for why they become part of a women's spiritual support group. Women seek to be part of a community that conducts rituals in a way that embraces our sense of ourselves as spiritual, that does justice, and that enhances our political sensibilities. These groups gather women who in a patriarchal culture must create the context of our own spirituality. They recognize the historical and contemporary oppression of women, especially poor women and women of diverse racial and ethnic backgrounds, and their dependent children. They seek to change social structures and personal attitudes to stop oppression. In these groups, ritual, therapy and justice interrelate as helpful components for feminist change.

FEMINIST RITUALS

Many feminist rituals are indebted to feminist groupwork and are informed by the principles of feminist therapy and feminist spirituality. They empower women for personal and social transformation. They offer women an important buffer to change, a way of consciously recognizing and supporting a life event rather than denying or rejecting it. They provide a collective place where women's ways of knowing–thinking, feeling, reacting and living–become normative. They focus on relationships that liberate and empower women who are moving from patriarchy to full humanity. They use symbols and stories, images and words, gestures and dances, along with a variety of art forms, which emerge from women's experiences. They value women's solidarity with one another and strengthen these bonds in community for overcoming violence in all its forms (Neu, 1993c, 1993d). They provide public occasions for remembering women's stories. They are intended to affect the behavioral, cognitive, and affective levels of participants.

Anthropologists Turner (1966) and van Gennep (1960) agree that ritual is prominent in all areas of uncertainty, anxiety, impotence, and disorder. Because rituals dramatize messages about continuity, predictability, and tradition they are inherently connective, providing integration of several kinds: (1) of the self with itself, as it contemplates change; (2) of the self with culture, by the use of common symbols; and (3) of the self with others, connecting celebrants into an often profound community. In ritual, doing is believing.

Rituals which mark transitions in the life cycle–rites of passage–are moments of dramatic teaching and socialization, occasions that societies construct to increase and clarify, to make their members most fully and deeply its own. Looking at traditional rites of passage, one quickly sees that there is a lack of rituals that mark women's life cycles. Feminists are creating new ceremonies of transition, like Sara's healing from childhood rape, Dolores' affirmation of a decision for abortion, Maria's celebration of coming out, Kathryn's integrating the daughter/mother relationship, Janet's affirming the wisdom of elderhood, and many more, such as menarche, reproductive choices and losses, infertility, career changes, healing, transition, relationship commitment, breaking of commitments, geographic uprooting, menopause, and death. Such rites of passage could teach women the meaning of our existence on women's terms. Feminist rituals celebrated in feminist spiritual support groups can assist the process of renewal and affirmation. The rituals marking Sara and Maria's turning points reveal this power.

DESCRIPTION OF SARA'S RITUAL– "BREAK THE UNHOLY SILENCE"

Sara's father, her perpetrator, had died within the year. His death was the catalyst for her, as she said, "to give myself the gift of integration and healing." She invited some of her friends, family and women from her survivors' group to gather in her home to mark this transition with her.

Her ritual began with a purification of her home to establish safety. Four women lit four candles to symbolize the collective power, tears, life and support of women. Sara's daughter invited participants to each take an evergreen branch and place them around the house to create a safe space for all of us. To begin a litany of healing I asked each woman to think of the anger and pain she experiences from violence, take a handkerchief from the basket, and tie a knot in it to symbolize her "no" to violence.

> We must be angry and scream, "No! No! No!" to the violence women and girls experience. To each violent act you hear, shout out "No! No! No!," raise the handkerchief over your head and pull the knot tight.
> To the men who harass women walking down the street, No! No! No!
> To fathers, brothers, grandfathers and uncles who sexually abuse girl-children,
> To husbands, lovers and partners who batter and rape their partners,
> To college men who rape their dates,
> To women who abuse their female lovers or partners,
> To whom else do we say no? Tell us and we will shout, No! No! No!

We then placed oil, an ancient symbol of strength and healing in many religious traditions, on one anothers' foreheads to invoke healing, saying to one another, "Reclaim your healing powers for yourself and for others."

Sara told her story about the terror and violence of her incest, named her wounds, read some of her poems, and put her father's knotted handkerchiefs in the center of the room to represent the tears of children, her tears. She then took scissors and cut the knots from the handkerchiefs. I invited the women to do the same with the handkerchiefs they used. Some women spontaneously untied the knots. Many of us wept. Sara proclaimed a litany of exorcism to which we responded, "Be gone! Be gone! Be gone!"

> I release the chronic pain of 45 years
> I release the pain in my jaws, my legs, my head, my entire body
> I release the pain of the selves who went into hiding
> I release the pain of searching for myself around the world
> I release the pain of disturbed intimate relationships
> I release the need to maintain silence about my incest

> I release the attachment to wanting my father's admission of raping me

Naming the different parts of Sara's personalities as she named them, the community responded:

> We restore to you, Sara, the innocence with which you were born and which was brutally stolen from you soon after your birth. We give thanks for all the intricate ways your selves have stayed hidden. We celebrate their coming out.
>> We welcome home Sue who remembers everything that happened . . .
>> We welcome home Studius, the obsessive compulsive student who studied hard to find a way out . . .
>> We welcome home Shelly who took care of her abusers to stay alive . . .
>> We welcome home Sewey the seamstress who kept creativity visible . . .

Sara then said: "All the split off selves choose reunion now . . . . "

We blessed Sara's home and work. We sang and danced. We wrote notes to Sara telling her how she is a blessing to us; we each called Sara's name, shared what we had written, and gave her the papers as a keepsake. To close, we passed the four candles around the circle and committed ourselves to breaking the cycle of violence, saying, "My sister, as long as your light burns, violence will be overcome."

Discussion of Sara's Ritual

Incest is shrouded with secrecy. Carrying such a secret inevitably breeds a sense of isolation, of being freakishly different, of being unspeakably dirty and shameful. In individual therapy, I struggle to convince the client who has survived incest that incest and child abuse occur frequently, even in epidemic proportions. A group automatically breaks the isolation experienced by incest survivors. In the feminist spiritual support group, Sara and the other women experienced emotional support, deepened their friendships, shared their spiritual journeys, and laughed and cried their way to health and healing.

According to Herman (1992), the core experiences of psychological trauma are disempowerment and disconnection from others. Recovery, therefore, is based upon the empowerment of the survivor and the creation of new connections. She states that recovery unfolds in three stages: the establishment of safety, remembrance and mourning, and reconnection with ordinary life.

Sara's ritual recognized these stages of recovery and added another dimension to it. Participants placed evergreen branches around the house to establish safety. Sara told the story of her trauma and mourned in the litany what was lost to her, what the incest destroyed. After integrating her split off selves, the ritual closed by reconnecting Sara to her ordinary life of home and work. Collectively, women named evil, rejected violent acts, and committed ourselves to break the cycle of violence. We offered one another support and healing in the context of a caring community. In blessing Sara we empowered and comforted her and ourselves. We restored her self-esteem and well-being as well as ours.

DESCRIPTION OF MARIA'S RITUAL: "COMING OUT: COMING HOME"

Maria, a Cuban-American clergywoman, had struggled through her coming out process. She invited lesbian and heterosexual friends from her women-church group and colleagues from her clergywomen's support group to her home to mark her awareness of identity, and to support her as a lesbian.

Her ritual began with friends creating a circle of care by speaking their names, acknowledging their support of Maria, and giving their hand to the person next to them as a sign of that empowerment. Four women blessed the four directions and elements of the universe–fire, air, water and earth–for "they have called home to the world our friend Maria."

(Blesser of Fire, South, lights a candle.)
Source of Fire, O Searing Flame,
Fill Maria's heart and all our hearts with the spark of passion.
Empower us and every lesbian, gay, bi-sexual and transgendered person with courage to emerge from cocoons of hiberna-

tion and isolation.
Release our imaginations from their hiding places.
Guiding Light, Fire of Justice, One Who brings Us Home.
Amen. Blessed be. Let it be so.

(Blesser of Air, East, plays wind chimes.)
    Source of Air, O Whispering Wind,
    Fill Maria's lungs and all our lungs with the breath of healing.
    Blow away the staleness.
    Bring freshness into our lives.
    Gentle Breeze, Rustling Sound, One Who brings Us Home.
    Amen. Blessed be. Let it be so.

(Blesser of Water, West, pours water into a bowl.)
    Source of Water, Ever-bubbling spring,
    Fill Maria's being and all our beings with emotions that flow
    freely.
    Wash away the hurts and pains of all oppressed people.
    Quench our thirst for spiritual and sexual connection.
    Ocean Womb, Wellspring of Life, One Who brings Us Home.
    Amen. Blessed be. Let it be so.

(Blesser of Earth, North, brings a basket of bread.)
    Source of Earth, Mother of Our Being,
    Fill Maria's body and all our bodies with courage for loving
    one another.
    Cradle and protect us as we discover our real selves.
    Enlighten us with dreams, visions and inner wisdom.
    Sacred Ground, Fertile Soil, One Who brings Us Home.
    Amen. Blessed be. Let it be so.

Maria told her story of coming out. Then participants thanked her for trusting us enough to share her experience with us. We honored her by giving her several mementos: the candle to symbolize her passion for truth, the wind chimes to symbolize the unique melody that is hers, the water bowl to represent the deep well that she is, and the basket of bread to symbolize the nourishment that she is to us and to others she meets.

We offered a "Litany of Thanksgiving" to praise Loving Wisdom for creating Maria a lesbian. To each phrase we responded, "We praise you."

> Loving Wisdom, we praise you for creating Maria a lesbian. We praise you for creating us your lesbian, gay, bisexual and transgendered people.
>> For bringing us out of our closets and into full life, we praise you.
>> For embracing us with your love and care,
>> For giving us a company of friends and a family of choice,
>> For teaching us that our sexuality is a gift for the community,
>> For strengthening us to cope with misunderstanding, fear, and hatred,
>> For helping us break through heterosexism and homophobia in ourselves, families and friends, culture and society, churches and synagogues,
>> For enlightening us with dreams of holy impatience,
>
> Loving Wisdom, we praise you for creating Maria a lesbian. We praise you for creating us your lesbian, gay, bisexual and transgendered people.

The ritual closed with blessing bread, wine and juice, eating a festive meal and embracing one another in love.

Discussion of Maria's Ritual

The experience of coming out to oneself is an important area about which therapists working with lesbians need to be knowledgeable. Women in the early stages of recognizing their lesbian identities are often terrified about the possibility of being lesbian. Women who are neither feminist nor lesbian-positive, and women who have had a narrow religious upbringing may harbor the secret suspicion that something is not quite right about them. Those who have suffered childhood sexual abuse may wonder if their childhood experience may have caused them to be a lesbian. Homophobia frightens most lesbians and causes many to become self-conscious and begin to question themselves. While some lesbians have an easier process, all break taboos.

Decisions about coming out to others are major ones for lesbians. Invisibility is disempowering. It means always having to be quiet about what is central in lesbian lives. It means living with the constant risk of unexpected exposure. Coming out can mean loss of jobs, family rejection, loss of friends, ridicule and violence. Coming out is nonetheless an assertion of self. It is the beginning of coming home to self. It is empowerment.

Cass (1979) cites six stages of coming out: identity confusion, identity comparison, identity tolerance, identity acceptance, identity pride, and identity synthesis.

Maria's ritual celebrates her coming out and being out. It affirms her identity acceptance, which is characterized by selective disclosure of sexual orientation. It empowers her to be able to face the times of self-doubt, the oppression of homophobia, and the injustice of prejudice. The gifts that Maria received during the ritual are transitional objects that remind her symbolically of the love and support of her friends. The blessing was empowering for all of us. The gifts, blessing and ritual strengthened her identity pride.

IMPLICATIONS FOR WOMEN AND THERAPY

Feminist critique has long held that women's voices need to be heard more powerfully, not only in the political arena, but in prose, poetry, ritual, art and human services as well. Feminist rituals have considerable power for women in therapy, for therapists, for women in feminist spiritual support groups and for society.

For women in therapy. Feminist rituals can empower women in therapy. They can offer women a collective spiritual support that marks their transitions, reduces their anxiety about changes to make these anxieties manageable, and empowers them to foster personal well-being and social transformation.

For therapists. Feminist rituals can empower therapists. They can be used in therapy sessions to promote empowerment of clients. Therapists can recommend that clients for whom spirituality is important participate in feminist spiritual support groups to connect them through networking and consciousness-raising about the experiences of women. Therapists can be empowered when we participate in our own rituals and feminist spiritual support groups.

For women in feminist spiritual support groups. Feminist rituals can empower women in feminist ritual support groups. They make it possible for women to retell women's stories and to recover feminist collective memories. Members of these groups can help each other become fully and critically aware of each other's situation as women. A life cycle ritual honoring a particular woman can remind others that a similar ritual is available to them and can inspire them to create one of their own.

For society. Feminist rituals can empower change in society. Life cycle rituals that mark women's rites of passage can empower society to pass on to future generations respect for women. They provide occasions for members of society to tell, listen to, pay attention to, and hear the stories of women's life cycles.

CONCLUSION

Feminist rituals have therapeutic potential for women who seek empowerment and healing. They have the capacity to ease difficult life transitions, to provide a lens for looking at relationships, to tap wellsprings of individual and joint creativity, to heal personal pain, to celebrate life, and to transform the political. Our therapy and our ritual, our spirituality and our politics must be interwoven so that with our impatience and our passion others can say of us, in the words of Judy Grahn (1977),

> . . . Many years back
> a woman of strong purpose
> passed through this section
> and everything else tried to follow.

REFERENCES

Budapest, Zsuzsanna E. (1989). *Grandmother of time.* New York: Harper & Row.
Butler, Sandra, & Wintram, Claire (1991). *Feminist groupwork.* Newbury Park, CA: Sage.
Cass, V. C. (1984). Homosexual identity formation: Testing a theoretical model. *Journal of Sex Research, 20,* 143-167.
Grahn, Judy. (1977). *The work of a common woman.* New York: St. Martin's Press.

Herman, Judith L. (1992). *Trauma and recovery.* New York: Basic.

Hunt, Mary E. (1990). Defining women-church. *WATERwheel, 3*(2), 1-3.

Miller, Jean Baker (1991b). Women and power. In Judith V. Jordan, Alexandra G. Kaplan, Jean Baker Miller, Irene P. Stiver, Janet L. Surrey (Eds.), *Women's growth in connection* (pp. 197-205). New York: Guilford.

Neu, Diann L. (1992). You are not alone. *WATERwheel, 4*(4), 4-5.

Neu, Diann L. (1993a). We are all daughters: Healing the daughter/mother relationship. *WATERwheel, 6*(1), 4-5.

Neu, Diann L. (1993b). Choosing wisdom: A croning ceremony. *WATERwheel, 6*(3), 4-5.

Neu, Diann L. (1993c). Women revisioning religious ritual. In Lesley A. Northrop (Ed.), *Women and religious ritual* (pp. 155-172). Washington, DC: The Pastoral Press.

Neu, Diann L. (1993d). Women-church transforming liturgy. In Marjorie Proctor-Smith and Janet Walton (Eds.), *Women at worship.* (pp. 163-178). Louisville, KY: Westminster/John Knox.

Neu, Diann L. & Hunt, Mary E. (1993). *Women-church sourcebook.* Silver Spring, MD: Waterworks Press.

Plaskow, Judith (1990). *Standing again at Sinai.* San Francisco: Harper and Row.

Ruether, Rosemary Radford (1985). *Women-church.* San Francisco: Harper & Row.

Schussler Fiorenza, Elisabeth (1983). *In memory of her.* New York: Crossroad.

Starhawk. (1982). *Dreaming the dark.* Boston: Beacon Press.

Surrey, Janet L. (1991). Relationship and empowerment. In Judith V. Jordan, Alexandra G. Kaplan, Jean Baker Miller, Irene P. Stiver, Janet L. Surrey (Eds.), *Women's growth in connection* (pp.162-180). New York: Guilford.

Turner, Victor (1966). *The ritual process.* Chicago: Aldine.

van Gennep, Arnold (1960). *The rites of passage.* Chicago: University of Chicago Press.

Winter, Miriam Therese, Stokes, Allison, & Lummis, Adair (1994). *Defecting in place: Women's claiming responsibility for their own spiritual lives.* New York: Crossroad.

Re-Membering Spirituality:
Use of Sacred Ritual in Psychotherapy

Anne R. Bewley

SUMMARY. Ritual has been used as a therapeutic tool within family therapy for nearly two decades. Our understanding of ritual has
been drawn from studies of cultures in which all life was viewed as
sacred. However, common use of ritual in therapy lifts ritual out of
its sacred context and secularizes it. Blending some of the key thinking in feminist theology with feminist psychology can help women
reconnect with a perspective on the sacred that is empowering. Reimbuing ritual with the sacred and expanding its use in therapy makes it
a powerful healing process for women.

"Ritual" is a word that has been in the psychotherapeutic vocabulary for nearly two decades as it has been used in family therapy as
a means of restructuring interactions and of marking events. This
use was extrapolated from the ways in which so-called primitive
cultures used ritual to articulate and reinforce their understanding of
life. While ritual originally served a sacred purpose in defining the

Anne R. Bewley received her PhD in psychology from The Union Institute in
1993. She is Director of Curriculum for Counseling Psychology at Antioch New
England Graduate School, 40 Avon Street, Keene, NH 03431-3516. A certified
clinical mental health counselor, Anne also maintains a small private practice in
Center Sandwich, NH, where she specializes in the treatment of women. The
theoretical foundation of her work lies in a synthesis of feminist spirituality,
feminist psychology, and psychosynthesis and her praxis as a Wiccan priestess.

[Haworth co-indexing entry note]: "Re-Membering Spirituality: Use of Sacred Ritual in Psycho-
therapy." Bewley, Anne R. Co-published simultaneously in *Women & Therapy* (The Haworth Press,
Inc.) Vol. 16, No. 2/3, 1995, pp. 201-213; and: *Women's Spirituality, Women's Lives* (ed: Judith Och-
shorn, and Ellen Cole) The Haworth Press, Inc., 1995, pp. 201-213; and: *Women's Spirituality, Women's
Lives* (ed: Judith Ochshorn, and Ellen Cole) Harrington Park Press, an imprint of The Haworth Press,
Inc., 1995, pp. 201-213. Multiple copies of this article/chapter may be purchased from The Haworth
Document Delivery Center [1-800-3-HAWORTH; 9:00 a.m. - 5:00 p.m. (EST)].

201

individual, the community, and the spiritual nature and context of both, this purpose has been dropped in our current applications of ritual to therapy, a setting and process commonly (and, I believe, falsely) seen as more secular than sacred.

The purpose of this paper is to discuss the value and process of reimbuing therapeutic ritual with the sacred. First, I will describe the nature of ritual and review the current uses of ritual in therapy. Following that review, I will discuss some of the trends in feminist theology which speak to the value of ritual for women. I will demonstrate some of the ways in which I have sought to combine the two, capitalizing on the uses of ritual in ways which specifically name the transformative process–i.e., therapy–as sacred. I will conclude by offering some guidelines for developing sacred ritual as well as some comments regarding the indications and contra-indications of its use.

THE NATURE OF RITUAL

Our use of ritual in therapy today is drawn from the work of social or cultural anthropologists. Ritual is seen as consisting of "stereotyped, symbolic acts or interactions" through which ideologies, values, and norms are expressed. Its purpose is to sanction or perpetuate a social system (van der Hart, 1983). Rituals consist of fixed patterns of acts which are specific to certain situations. These patterns occur throughout the culture, although they may occur only once in each individual's life. They are prescribed by the society and include binding implicit and explicit instructions as to their indications and use. Symbolic objects, acts, or words, the "building blocks of ritual," are used to convey meaning on several different levels. This "multivocality" carries messages directly to the unconscious, instigating changes in consciousness.

In so-called primitive societies, the needs of the individual are met through the survival and prosperity of the group. Individual and communal rituals serve to bring order to the multiplicity of relationships within a society by inducting individuals into that society and supporting them in being cooperative, contributing members of the group throughout the life cycle. In addition to safeguarding social structure, rituals have a physiological and psychological effect on the culture. By providing an explanation of the relationships between individuals, their society, and the natural world, rituals help people resist chaos and empower them to act appropriately.

There are several types of ritual which prevail in indigenous cultures. These include rites of transition, rites of continuity, and rites of healing. Rites of transition are designed to mark the passage from one stage of life to another. Rites of continuity have to do with welcoming new members, terminating relationships, and intensifying the sense of belonging and cohesiveness within a group. Rites of healing are used to restore ecological unity within a group when it is threatened by conflict, tension, or disintegration. It is the use of rituals to support and balance a culture's structure, to aid in its function, and to heal its wounds that makes ritual so appealing to family therapists (van der Hart, 1983).

As anthropology meets psychology, there is a debate as to whether ritual is essentially a religious or a social phenomenon. As all societies create rituals, so they also create theologies. One early definition of ritual stated explicitly that ritual has "reference to beliefs in mystical beings or powers" (Turner, 1967, cited in Imber-Black, Roberts, & Whiting, 1988). This clause was deleted from later uses of this definition as it was noted that anthropologists worked in cultures in which all life and all life activities were seen as sacred. Rather than bringing this attitude of sacredness along with the concept of ritual, however, therapists employing ritual in their work tend to perpetuate the prevailing cultural (i.e., Christian) perspective that separates secular and sacred and to focus only on the more secular applications of the concept. "Sacred" has been reduced to "special" as ritual is used to mark, name, or set apart a secular (non-sacred) process.

USES OF RITUAL IN FAMILY THERAPY

Ritual was introduced to family therapy by Maria Selvini Palazzoli and her colleagues in 1974. It was further developed through the work of Onno van der Hart. These and other clinicians discovered that the concept of ritual provided a new source of inspiration in facilitating change within the family "society," and the concept was quickly adopted by strategic family therapists.

Evan Imber-Black (1988) noted five themes which serve to orient the use of ritual in therapy: membership, healing, identity, belief expression and negotiation, and celebration. These themes are part of any family's normative functioning in daily life, times of celebration, and life cycle transitions. As such, they provide a ground from which to work with a client or clients through the process of restructuring interactions, reworking emotional material, and facilitating change.

The use of ritual is indicated whenever a family is experiencing difficulty in making transitions or when it is in crisis and needs healing. It is seen as a creative adjunct to "normal therapy." In implementing ritual, the therapist identifies a key symbol which holds the condensed meaning of the transition or crisis. He or she then assigns a set of actions around that symbol and prescribes that set to the family or individual. The ritual is given a solemn or dramatic tinge by being different, unusual, set apart from the rest of the therapeutic encounter.

THEMES IN FEMINIST THEOLOGY

While the largest body of critical study in feminist theology has been in the area of Christianity, Judaism has also come under feminist scrutiny, and there is an emerging feminist critique of Buddhism. In recent years, the critique of traditional, patriarchal frames of reference has been expanded to incorporate the voices of feminists from many cultures and ethnic traditions. Under the larger umbrella of feminist spirituality, a wide variety of perspectives, including Wiccan (and other neo-pagan), African, African-Caribbean, and Native American world-views, speak to women about empowering and healing themselves and each other, building supportive communities, and connecting or reconnecting with the sacred as the context of daily life.

Christianity has been most influential in the construction of the cultural, social, and intellectual foundations of Western society. Thus, I will use the feminist critique of Christianity to provide an example of the ways in which spiritual frames of reference that are grounded in patriarchy can be reviewed, reconstructed, revised, or relinquished to provide a healthy alternative perspective for women. It is important to remember, however, that the critique of Christianity serves as only one source of the revolutionary and empowering themes found in feminism and which speak to all women who seek liberation.

The feminist critique of Christianity has been approached from two main perspectives. There are those who seek to reform the religion from within and those who see the only possibilities for change as lying without. In the first category are such theologians as Elisabeth Schüssler Fiorenza and Rosemary Radford Ruether.

Fiorenza (1983) undertook a feminist theological reconstruction of Christian history in which she highlighted the social and cultural movements of the early church, the role women and other oppressed people played in those movements, and the systematic repression of equality that occurred in the first several centuries after the crucifixion. She pulled apart the weave of the androcentric texts to inspect and find meaning in the spaces between the threads, thus reconstructing history to show women as central figures in both the Jesus movement and the early Christian church. Viewing women's experience as fundamental to theological understanding, Fiorenza removed the patriarchy from the center of Christianity.

Fiorenza pointed out that women's religious communities have always existed within the church in spite of the efforts of the male hierarchy to bring them under its control. With an established tradition of women's leadership and importance in the history of the church behind them, women today can acknowledge their own spiritual power and gifts. Claiming these communities of women and their history as women's heritage is a way of rejecting the patriarchal structures that oppress, limit, and divide women in the church.

Rosemary Radford Ruether (1984) provided a critique of Christian theology and explored its compatibility with feminism. From her perspective, there must be a change in both church and society. It is not enough to withdraw from traditional Christianity and form an alternative community. Change must begin with weeding out the roots of sexism in the established church in order for there to be any meaningful and lasting change in society.

On the other side of this feminist debate are those who feel that the Christian church is a lost cause as far as women's rights and psychological and spiritual well-being are concerned. They see the road to spiritual and cultural wellness as bypassing, rather than traversing or reforming, the traditional church. Here we find the voices of Naomi Goldenberg and Carol Christ.

Goldenberg (1979) described the death of the Father God as a necessary consequence of rising feminism. A psychologist of religion and feminist theologian, Goldenberg critiqued the role psychology and religion have played in fostering oppression. She articulated the need for more affirming models and sacred symbols for women and described feminist Wicca as a means of helping women reach an understanding of the Goddess as a more life-giving source of strength.

Moving from the institutional to the personal, theologian Carol Christ (1986) explored the themes of women's spiritual experience. Because Christian texts are based on men's experience, she highlighted the telling of women's stories and spiritual experiences as a way in which women are able to understand and change their lives and their world. Rather than affirming one universal spirituality, Christ stated that spiritual meaning occurs in the unique experiences women have. While women may share experiences and needs that they can meet in community, Christ viewed spirituality as an individual, rather than collective experience. She found fault with the emphasis in traditional theological scholarship on universal truths, as proclamations of such truths devalue knowledge and faith gained from personal understanding, reflection, and experience.

Much of the richness of the feminist critique of Christianity lies in the example it provides and the directions to which it points in finding healthy alternatives for women both inside and outside their "churches of origin." Liberation, community, a desire to return to the earth and our bodies, the value of symbols as tools of creation and change, and the importance of personal experience as a source of knowledge and understanding are themes that emerge from this critique (and others) that speak to women of many faiths. Women are encouraged to inspect their belief systems and forms of worship for those threads and patterns in the tapestry of religion that portray their positive involvement in a church of choice. They are asked to go back to the beginning of formal religions for early messages of equality and liberation. They are also encouraged to step outside of the frames that have bound their perspective for alternative points of view, for images of the sacred that are not patriarchally based. For many women, this has meant turning to an understanding of God as Goddess and finding within the modern pagan and earth-based traditions forms of worship and expressions of faith that are more holistic and inclusive than those they experienced within their former churches.

Both within and outside of traditional churches, women are finding images and forms which foster their empowerment, self-expression, and desire for community. They are learning to support one another in spiritual and communal growth in an active way. They are finding new symbols for this growth and using those symbols in sacred rituals to heal themselves and others, shape inner experience, transform perceptions, and structure new forms of connection with self, others, and the sacred.

THERAPY AT THE CROSSROAD

In ritual, we come to a point where feminist psychology and theology can meet. While the use of ritual in psychotherapy has, for the most part, been viewed and described as secular, I believe there is enormous healing power in reimbuing ritual with the sacred, re-membering spirituality and the healing process in an intentional and clearly articulated way. Ritual sprang from societies in which all life was considered holy. Rather than continuing to remove ritual from the sacred to fit our view of therapy as a secular process (and perpetuate a false dichotomy), we can shift our point of view in therapy to see our work as holy.

One obvious question is that regarding the nature of the difference between secular and sacred ritual. At times, it is clear; and at other times, the difference is subtle and has more to do with the frame around the experience, the context in which ritual is placed, and the attitude with which it is engaged or exercised. From the perspective of strategic therapy, ritual is developed by the therapist who, sometimes, but not always, solicits the ideas of the client. It is prescribed as a form of treatment by the therapist which is "taken" by the client. Van der Hart (1983) discussed the difficulty of motivating clients to engage in prescribed ritual and described means through which therapists can become attuned to the symbols and representational systems of their clients in order to make ritual a more desired task.

From my perspective, sacred ritual is a cooperative process. It is a form of intervention which is, perhaps, suggested by the therapist but which is always co-created by the client and the therapist. Together, therapist and client explore the client's understanding of spirituality. Finding an experience that she can embrace, they then identify the key symbols in which the experience may be condensed and formulate the appropriate symbolic acts. While the therapist may take the lead out of her greater experience with the process, the client is the "celebrant" at the ritual. Sacred ritual is framed in the context of the holy. Therapist and client name the work that is to be done as a sacred process, one in which the presence of the sacred is expressly acknowledged. The space in which the ritual is to be conducted is cleansed and set apart for the work, and Spirit, in a form determined by the client and her belief system, remembered in that space. The work is done with the intention of healing, but without attachment to outcome. As ritual is a cooperative and creative process, it is never prescribed, and since it emerges from the desire of the client and the suggestion of the therapist, motivation is not an issue I have encountered. Thus, while on the surface secular and sacred ritual may look quite the same, they are founded on a different premise and operate in different contexts.

CASE EXAMPLES

Let me give you a couple of examples from my own work which illustrate the ways in which sacred ritual can be implemented within therapy.

Paula is a 48 year old woman who was working on relationship issues. She was brought up Catholic, a faith she abandoned as a young woman. She is now drawn by Native American spiritual practices. Before Christmas, Paula fell into a depression which took a toll on her relationship with her partner because she did not feel up to joining in the festivities. She had tried to focus on the Winter Solstice as a seasonal marker and time of change, but found her meditations interrupted by memories of loss and grief. As we explored this, she told me that as a child, it had been her custom to help her father trim the Christmas tree, thus kicking off the holiday season. When he had died six years ago, she had been actively engaged in addiction. It became apparent that her grieving process was incomplete. As part of our work together, we created a ritual through which Paula could honor her father by trimming the tree with him once again.

Later that week, she cleaned the living room, smudging it with herbs that held a special meaning to her. She then created an ancestor altar near the neglected Christmas tree. She arranged a picture of her father, some of his special things she had inherited, and candles and incense, put on some of his favorite music, and sat quietly near the altar and the tree with her drum–her own sacred object. She drummed herself softly into trance, welcoming the presence of the spirit guides whom she felt watched over her path. Into this meditative place, she invoked the spirit of her father and felt his presence. She spoke with him a while, sharing her feelings of guilt about not having been present at his death, of missing him now, and of wishing for a sense of connection with him which transcended death. She wept and felt comforted–and proceeded to trim the tree with him.

As she told me about this the next week, it was clear that something had shifted deep within her. She seemed at peace. What had been an empty space was filled with the sense of connection she had sought. Since then, she has spoken to me of feeling her father's spirit guiding her at times of indecision and uncertainty.

This ritual came after a considerable amount of "talk therapy." It provided a missing piece–an experience of forgiveness and connection that we had not been able to access in any other way. Paula's work freed up a considerable amount of emotional energy which she reinvested in her relationship with her partner. While there have been many things that influenced her healing, she felt strongly that this ritual marked the turning point for her.

My work with Maddy provides another example. Maddy was having considerable difficulty getting over the loss that occurred when her partner moved out-of-state. Although the couple was estranged at the time of her partner's move, Maddy still felt a deep connection that was laden with jealousy, guilt, and anger. We spent many sessions working on these feelings, but they persisted.

As Maddy is drawn to Goddess-based images and forms, I asked her if she would be interested in creating a healing ritual. It took several sessions to negotiate the process, as my question helped her realize that there was a part of her that was not interested in getting over the feelings she was having as they enabled her to stay connected–albeit painfully. After a particularly bad week full of hateful, rageful cross-country phone calls, she agreed that she needed to release the situation.

We planned the ritual together. Maddy agreed to make a small doll to represent the part of her that held her feelings of jealousy, guilt and anger. The doll was to have a pocket of some sort into which Maddy could put small things. In our next session, we lit some candles and described the room as sacred space, invoking into it the spirit of healing. Then, I asked Maddy to sit with her doll in the center of the room and to allow her feelings to come up as she listened to the music. I rocked with her, attuning to her movement, as she cried. Next, I asked her to dance with her doll as she listened to the song once again. Again, I attuned to her movement noting that her feet remained rooted in place. She was stuck.

We sat for a while to process what was occurring. In the middle of our discussion, she looked sharply at her doll and said, "These aren't my feelings about Andrea. This doll is about me! What I'm missing is me!" At that point, I asked her to dance once again, this time holding her doll as if it were all the parts of herself that she felt were missing or alienated. The music played, and Maddy danced around the room, moving freely through the available space. As I mirrored her movement, I joined her sense of freedom and life and joy.

Following her dance, Maddy set about making a set of "Maddy Cards," naming and affirming one of her qualities on each small card. She stuck these cards into the doll's apron pocket with the intention of drawing one each time she felt tempted to reach out to someone else for a part of herself. Since that time, Maddy has been able to let go of her partner and see the separation as a necessary time for her to attend to the process of reclaiming, appreciating, and nurturing herself.

These two examples–particularly the last one–could be described as gestalt-based, expressive therapy sessions, and they do include elements of both those treatment approaches. What makes them different is the fact that the activity involved is named as sacred and healing and is placed in a frame that supports it as such. The work of the ritual is imbued not only with the meaning the individual brings to the experience, but the power of the sacred, as well. While I believe that the sacred is always present, especially where there is healing, naming that presence as such seems another important feature of this work–and one which, again, distinguishes it from a fancy Gestalt or elaborate expressive therapy technique.

GUIDELINES, INDICATIONS, AND CONTRA-INDICATIONS

As a form, sacred ritual need not have a rigid structure. Basically, there are three parts to any ritual: a beginning, a middle, and an end. The beginning involves preparing the celebrant and space and naming that space and the work to be done as sacred. The middle has to do with the "work" of the ritual, whatever task is being done, and the end consists of closing the work and releasing the space. I almost always suggest adding to the work of the ritual some way of grounding that work in the "real world." Thus, the heart of the work occurs symbolically during the ritual and through an actual act in the world following it. In Maddy's case, for example, we agreed that she would draw a "Maddy card" each morning and create an affirmation from that word to use during the day. She was also to consult with her doll for advice whenever she felt the compulsion to call her ex-partner.

The work of the ritual can take many forms. It always involves a symbolic object, act or word. One can burn, bury, wash, cut, tie, make, take apart, fold, imagine, affirm, denounce, name, and will. It is important for the client to work within her belief system. For some women, that may mean using the symbols, intent, and process of the Christian sacramental forms of baptism, confession, communion, marriage, and burial. However, other cultural traditions provide ideas for rituals which can serve as sources of inspiration, and those familiar and comfortable with rituals from other cultures can respectfully adopt those forms.

Rituals can be adapted for use with almost any population. I have found it particularly effective in work with women recovering from addiction and/or trauma. It is also useful as a tool in therapy for women with mood and anxiety disorders. It is important to remember, however, that in working with ritual, we are working with symbols, and the impact of symbols on the unconscious mind is powerful. For that reason, I am guarded in suggesting ritual work for clients with poor ego strength. If I do suggest ritual work with these clients, I emphasize the importance of form and structure and work to keep the ritual as concrete as possible. Tying a string around a celebrant's wrist as a reminder that she is entitled to boundaries might be one symbolic act that could work well with a boundary-disordered client. Doing more abstract work with imagery, an experience which can be frightening with someone who has difficulty determining where she ends and someone else begins, is not indicated. Ritual work with clients who are thought disordered and who otherwise have a poor ability to ground in reality is contra-indicated.

There are several caveats that apply. The first has to do with clients who have experienced ritual abuse. I have found that the kind of work I am describing is very useful in helping these women heal. However, for them, the term "ritual" is a loaded one which can evoke intrusive memories. I have had to find another way to describe and frame our work, calling it a ceremony or celebration and avoiding the use of the word "ritual" until it can be seen in a positive, healing light. I also remind these women of the power of their role as celebrant. *They* are directing the process, not someone else. It is within *their* power to heal through a form once used to wound. This corrective recapitulation, itself, is healing.

The second caveat has to do with the idea of destruction. I will not suggest or participate in rituals in which a client wishes to destroy or otherwise harm any aspect of herself or someone else. There is an ethic in Wicca that holds that whatever goes around comes around thricefold. I always ask my clients if they are willing to receive back the work they are doing. Thus, when helping a client overcome her fear of a jealous ex-partner, we do not focus on binding that ex-partner, but on empowering the celebrant. In facilitating the release of dysfunctional behaviors, we do not cut off the offending part of the self, but provide it with alternative nourishment, attention, and inclusion within the personality in exchange for assistance in eradicating the unwanted behaviors. Symbols and symbolic acts are potent. It may seem like "nothing" to write a sexual abuse perpetrator's name on a piece of paper and cut that paper into tiny bits to be flushed away, but doing so may nourish, rather than wash away, seeds of hatred. It is far better to write a letter of rage, cut it up and flush it, and engage in a ritual of purification and self-renewal. "If it harms no one, do what you will." Otherwise, beware of the rule of three.

CONCLUSION

The process I have described here is both simple and complex. Sacred ritual can serve to heal, to empower, and to change consciousness and behavior. In my experience, a ritual that is carefully constructed between client and therapist will further the work of "ordinary" therapy. The role of the therapist is to help the client reconnect with an understanding and experience of the sacred that works for her and to implement that experience into the therapeutic setting.

REFERENCES

Christ, Carol P. (1980). *Diving deep and surfacing: Women's writing on spiritual quest.* (2nd ed.). Boston: Beacon Press.

Fiorenza, Elisabeth S. (1983). *In memory of her: A feminist theological reconstruction of Christian origins.* New York: Crossroads Press.

Goldenberg, Naomi R. (1979). *Changing of the gods: Feminism and the end of traditional religions.* Boston: Beacon Press.

Imber-Black, Evan; Roberts, Janine; & Whiting, Richard. (Eds.). (1988). *Rituals in families and family therapy.* New York: W. W. Norton.

Ruether, Rosemary R. (1983). *Sexism and God-talk: Toward a feminist theology.* Boston: Beacon Press.

Van der Hart, Onno (1983). *Rituals in psychotherapy: Transition and continuity.* (Angie Pleit-Kuiper, trans.). New York: Irvington Publishers.

Explorations of the Unrecognized Spirituality of Women's Communion

Ellen B. Kimmel
Barbara W. Kazanis

SUMMARY. The spiritual dimensions of gatherings of women, particularly those with a dedication to something beyond the self, are explored. Women's groups are argued to be a potentially valuable resource for therapy as they provide a safe place where the "feminine principle" can be honored and reclaimed. The paper employs an experiential learning model and uses stories to illustrate key points. Storytelling as prayer is analyzed as a vehicle for healing, developing, and transformation within each woman and the larger community. Three types of stories–Medicine, Teaching and Stories of Power–are described along with three supportive functions women's groups play.

A way of conceptualizing the distinctiveness of feminist therapy (and feminist pedagogy) is that its purpose is to heal the last 2500

Ellen B. Kimmel, Professor of Education and Psychology, and former Department Chair and Dean, University of South Florida (USF), is Past President of Division 35 (Psychology of Women) of the American Psychological Association and a longtime feminist activist. Barbara W. Kazanis, Associate Professor of Arts Education and Director of the Arts and Human Development Institute, USF, is a practicing artist and a certified Expressive Arts Therapist.

Ellen Kimmel may be written at University of South Florida, 4202 East Fowler Avenue, FAO 100U, Rm. 268, Tampa, FL 33620-7750.

[Haworth co-indexing entry note]: "Explorations of the Unrecognized Spirituality of Women's Communion." Kimmel, Ellen B., and Barbara W. Kazanis. Co-published simultaneously in *Women & Therapy* (The Haworth Press, Inc.) Vol. 16, No. 2/3, 1995, pp. 215-227; and: *Women's Spirituality, Women's Lives* (ed: Judith Ochshorn, and Ellen Cole) The Haworth Press, Inc., 1995, pp. 215-227; and: *Women's Spirituality, Women's Lives* (ed: Judith Ochshorn, and Ellen Cole) Harrington Park Press, an imprint of The Haworth Press, Inc., 1995, pp. 215-227. Multiple copies of this article/chapter may be purchased from The Haworth Document Delivery Center [1-800-3-HAWORTH; 9:00 a.m. - 5:00 p.m. (EST)].

215

years' wounding of the feminine principle (Woodman, 1992; Simpkinson, 1992). Women through the ages have been ravaged in the very cells of their bodies. They were and still are shamed, degraded, victimized (Goodman, Koss, & Russo, 1993), silenced and filled with self doubt. Those who resisted were shunned, shackled, cloistered, or burned at the stake. Driven and redefined by negative masculine values, women have been disconnected from their bodies and souls. As therapists, teachers and friends, we search for processes that re-weave mind, heart, body and behavior.

The basic purpose of this paper is to point to women's gatherings as a critical, powerful, and largely unused resource in binding this 2500-year-old wound. We contend that examination of the spirituality of women's groups, particularly those with a feminist consciousness or a dedication to something beyond the self, can illuminate experiential practices that will repair the dis-eases that affect women, disconnection, hunger, abuse, neglect and violence.

Today, women assemble in clinics, classrooms and kitchens to analyze patriarchy and tell their "soul" stories in order to regain their essence. These stories are told from a deep place of survival and life-force. As each story is shared, the others "settle into their bodies and become fully present," much like children snuggling down for bedtime stories. Voices are found and become stronger, individuated, accompanied by visible signs of growth reflected in a straightening of the spine or release of tension or, more dramatically, by a change of partner, job, or release from addiction.

Through the vehicle of this collaborative construction of her story, the "overtamed" or oversocialized woman (Estes, 1992) begins to claim her birth right and trust her instincts, body, authentic expressiveness and power. Therapeutically, blame shifts from inside to the social world outside. Shame and doubt begin to diminish. While these events describe in part the formal, deliberate work of therapists and teachers, they equally fit what transpires in other, less formal, meetings of women, from professional or activist conferences to "deep lunches." Something "more than" occurs, something nourishing that feeds the "soul famine" within and heals the spirit. Our step is bouncier, spirits raised.

To make our message personally meaningful to the reader, we ask that you recall your formal and informal times with other women, coffees, walks and all forms of intimate talks. Barbara calls this "profundity on the run," in contrast to spiritual practice through retreat. Jill Nelson (1993) speaks of "homegirls," the ones in our lives with whom we share it all. Through resonation and reverberation you can transform this unconscious experience into useable understandings to inform your practice and teaching. The Lewinian learning cycle as elaborated by Kolb (1984) is one way to analyze the processes that occur when women come together and is the model we will follow in this paper. In the experiential learning model, one begins with a Concrete Activity, in this case the acts of assembling and storytelling (or recollection of same) with their concomitant feelings of excitement, arousal, delight, anticipation. The second stage consists of "publishing the data" or talking about the concrete experience, that is, describing what happened and how we react to it. This phase is called "Reflective Observation" and is deemed critical in individuals' learning (changing) anything from their experience. From all the data offered by group members who share the experience, a search for meaning, for patterns and relationships, ensues. This is the third stage called Abstract Conceptualization. Finally, through Active Experimentation new concepts, insights, lessons, and/or meanings are taken "outside" the learning community where individuals further test them and revise them. The cycle continues. (See Figure 1.)

Let's begin with a story, one offered by Valerie Macleod (October, 21, 1993), a therapist and a doctoral student of Ellen's.

Valerie worked with a group of low SES women mandated by the courts to participate in group therapy. Despite initial resistance to the entire notion of talking about problems to strangers, once the first woman ventured her story, the dam broke and the group began to "happen." Valerie's comment was that she felt privileged to be a

FIGURE 1. Hindu labyrinth. Penetration of inner mysteries.

part of their process, awed at what they accomplished. In their last session, as the participants expressed what the experience meant to them, one woman said it all in terms of this paper. "Coming to our meetings for me was just like going to church, except that instead of worshiping the god out there, I worshiped the god in me."

Elinor Gadon (1992) noted that before we can evolve as mature professionals, we must identify our own experience of the sacred and feel that experience is validated. Many other feminists also feel that, in the exploration of women's spirituality, lies " . . . the leading edge for the healing of our culture into a more just society, a place where women and men can find wholeness in an integration of mind, body and spirit" (Gadon, 1992, p. 79).

One working definition of spiritual is Chopra's (1993) " . . . spirit is wholeness, the continuity of awareness that oversees all the bits and pieces of awareness" (p. 37). Berne and Savory (1991) offer, "Spirituality is my way of being, acting, relating, thinking, and choosing in light of my ultimate values" (p. 73). Spiritual growth demands healing and working toward wholeness, our own, our intimates' and the larger community's. The spiritual aspects of healing are often defined as "a single moment of knowing that you are connected to every other thing on earth and beyond" (Achterberg, 1993, p. 48). Important to add is that the World Health Organization has defined illness and disease as "a rupture in life's harmony."

Some, such as Mary Daly, are attempting to re-vision harmony through new images of God that are genderless, and others, like Jean Shinoda Bolen or Gloria Orenstein, are reactivating the "goddess movement" in their explorations (Ress, 1993). We identify with that even-harder-to-document strain of women who are carefully constructing a spiritual life from a confluence of sources. All three strands share the search to (1) discard language that oppresses; (2) find images that will inspire us; (3) see ultimate values in terms of needs and hungers that arise at various junctures in our development and (4) effect cultural transformation. Scholarship, activism, and the practice of therapy must be accompanied by other processes less tangible, less obvious, for these four to occur. We must create new narratives, using intuition, imagination, memory, foresight and vision (Orenstein, 1990). And we suggest that is exactly the spiritual work that goes on in women's groups. (See Figure 2.)

FIGURE 2. Greek dancing women.

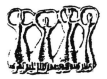

We are social creatures. Lacking participation in groups, we wither and die. Groups provide social support to enhance material and psychological well-being, encouragement, acceptance, and caring (Johnson & Johnson, 1991). Social bonding occurs when we perceive that others are like us and they reciprocate. Any group can become spiritual, but *not every group* is spiritual. What makes a group spiritual is "sharing a larger self, an interconnected self" (Chopra, 1993, p. 56). Indigenous cultures have always understood this.

Indigenous people had natural meeting places in the fires around which they sat and talked spontaneously at a very deep level. Contemporary women have no fires and are struggling to create such natural meeting places. Yet, women create their own version of the fireplace where the transmission of wisdom occurs through shared visions and the oral tradition of storytelling. The re-activation of traditional wisdom enables women to reconnect with their primary natural instincts (the Wild Woman). Clarissa Pinkola Estes (1992), a current spokesperson of this tradition and cantadora (keeper of stories), said, "How does Wild Woman affect women? With Wild Woman as ally, as leader, model, teacher . . . [she] carries the bundles for healing; she carries everything a woman needs to be and know. She carries the medicine for all things. She carries stories and dreams and words and songs and signs and symbols" (p. 12). We hope to convince you, reader, that women's groups function as a circle around the fire–that they allow women to reconnect with their original goodness by providing rituals, multivocal symbols, the finding of voice, and the unfolding of stories. We argue that they grant a sense of dignity, place, and harmonized, connected purpose. (See Figure 3.)

FIGURE 3. Western archaic bell signifying the arrival of the spirit.

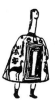

Feminist storytelling has helped us to:

1. expand our history to include feminine aspects of divinity;
2. point to new understandings of our physical and spiritual connections as humans to each other and the Natural World;
3. become open to the consideration of energies, powers, wisdom, that we generally refer to as spiritual, magical, Shamanic, or intuitive, as real and causally effective (Stone, 1990).
4. deal with the spiritual or mystical aspects of internal and external realities to help change our lives.

Those tales, legends, myths that contain all the instruction needed for her psychic development comprise "a woman's soul drama" (Estes, 1992, p. 15). As a presentational art form, stories offer " . . . the knife of insight, the flame of the passionate life, the breath to speak what one knows, the courage to stand what one sees without looking away, the fragrance of the wild soul" (Estes, 1992, p. 21). Since the spiritual resides in the details of life, telling one's personal or communal story authentically is a spiritual event.

In women's groups stories may serve as prayer and storytelling as ritual enactment. The story is a living presence which makes itself felt. It is visceral. One can be swept away with its energy. A sense of wonder is awakened when we ask, "How am I me?" Exploring this is a spiritual quest because it entails an investigation of one's place in the chain of life. Through stories we find our roots and insight into our purpose in existing (Simpkinson & Simpkinson, 1992).

We have identified at least three major types of stories–Medicine, Teaching and Stories of Power–that women recount when they come together. Medicine stories enter the psyche and act as a pharmacopeia to combat psychological malaise, requiring only that one listen. Traditional Hindu medical practice uses stories to heal (e.g., Skultans, 1991). The flow of images in stories is a similar medicine to listening to the ocean. They act as "antibiotic" that finds the source of the infection and concentrates there, that is, straight to the unconscious where they stir a deep authentic part of oneself. As medicine, they "close the wound that will not cease its bleeding," repair and reclaim lost parts of ourselves, our vitality or instinct (Estes, 1993). They enable prisoners and slaves and victims to bear suffering and maintain the will to live. Achterberg (1993) noted the accumulating data about the fact that women cancer patients who participate in groups live twice as long as those who do not gather in circles and share their stories. When medicine and healing are defined as including restoring harmony among the parts of our lives, the use of the story becomes the venue of therapy. Boyd-Franklin (1991) and Davies (1985) have already argued for the importance of women's groups to support therapy with African-American women. We feel it is crucial to all groups of women.

Teaching stories are embedded with instruction for living our lives. They re-educate us to our higher values and the necessity of embodying our spirits. Through them we can enter "the sacred" in everyday life where mind, heart and action are aligned. Teaching stories show us how to speak with our own voices, how to reach into the soft metaphorical parts of ourselves and how to extract wisdom for being and growing.

Consider the following story from a woman's full moon meditation group that has been meeting for 12 years.

A grandmother brings her granddaughter for a special ceremony of transition to puberty and menstruation. Each member blesses the young woman, welcomes her, and shares a story of the joy, surprise, mystery, or suffering of the first pains of menstruation. The celebration ends with songs of ancient and modern women, drumming, dancing and the eating of fruit, champagne and cakes.

Many feminists' stories are teaching stories, and first-person narratives are the cornerstone of many women's studies courses (e.g., Frankenberg, 1993). Through the experience of reading stories, students learn about groups and times other than their own. Feminist scholars have begun the task of providing "her-story" for students to learn from (Lerner, 1986).

Woodman and Estes have used stories to mobilize women's creative expression to heal and learn. Bolen (1993a) represents the movement interested in women's forging a political place for themselves, using Stories of Power to lead us to action in the world.

Consider the power of the Mothers of the Plaza, who, by simply becoming witness, helped bring down the terrorist regime which had caused the disappearance of thousands of their children in the 70s. At a time when all public demonstrations were forbidden, they walked every Thursday in a slow-moving circle around the Square holding posters with pictures and names of their missing children. When forbidden to meet in the plaza, they met silently in churches. Some lit candles, some prayed while passing notes. Decisions were made without a word spoken aloud.

Rather than chronicling what *is*, Power stories imagine reality, that is, expression begets beings. The story of the courageous Mothers of the Plaza inspired women in other countries, such as El Salvador and Guatemala, to take similar action. Power stories demand an answer to the question of the kind of reality we want to bring forth. They call for re-inventing the world. Indeed, feminist groups are collaboratively constructing new stories, new visions of human existence. Not only are they uncovering their personal ultimate values, but they are telling tales of power that illuminate ultimate values for humanity and invent a new cosmology (Diamond & Orenstein, 1990). (See Figure 4.)

Having entered the discussion of the spiritual dimension of women's groups through storytelling, we wish to mention three

FIGURE 4. American Indian symbol of potentially dangerous powers of the renewal of life.

other functions we discerned they serve that have spiritual qualities: (1) as a vessel for the members' stories; (2) as a vehicle for mentoring; and (3) as a safe place for the sacred to be acknowledged and celebrated.

Marion Woodman (1993), a spokesperson for the quest for the universal feminine voice, views the role of the therapist as a vessel, a container of her client's story, one who holds it and resonates to it. Bolen (1993b) has argued that one of the major functions of a friend or a therapist is being a witness to the life story of another person. However, many have noted that there are certain wounds that must be healed in groups, which must become the vessel or witness. For example, Brown and Zietfert (1988) stated that sexual violence and victimization disrupt connection to community. Thus, healing must necessarily involve reconnection to community through working in groups.

Lee (1989) described a psychology of women class where victims found affirmation and solidarity as they spoke and read from journals their stories of shame. Resnick-Sannes (1991) and others (e.g., Kreidler & England, 1990) claim that shame can only be dissolved in groups. The vessel (group) must be large and strong enough to hold the voicing of pain and wise enough to help place the blame for personal violation away from the individual and onto a lethal heritage of woman's body as evil and deserving of its victimization (Walden, 1992). Nelson (1991) had incest survivors make public presentations of their stories. Women in groups play the role of witness.

As Isabel Allende (1993) recounted, I had the mission of being a witness 20 years ago, and that changed my life forever. I, along with other journalists in Chile during the military coup in 1973, decided to be witnesses of the events. Although we could not publish the information, we had to remember what was happening. Everything I had witnessed was inside me like a heavy load without accomplishing what I needed to do–tell the world what had happened. Being a witness is my mission in the world and this is what I do when I tell stories.

Alice Walker (1993) agreed with Allende saying, "If you're in a situation in which something horrible is happening and spirit is being crushed, if you can't do anything else, you can witness it.

That is something you do in your role as storyteller." She said of her book about genital mutilation, "If nothing else, I say that I know these children are suffering, these women are in pain. I think there is power in that." The artist Sarah Teofanov created a T-shirt that read, "I Am Your Witness," for girls and women being raped in Sarajevo (Howa, 1993).

A second function of groups is to foster mentors and the act of mentoring. In ancient times teaching was a process of direct transmission of wisdom that emerged from deep rapport. It was referred to as "from mouth to ear" (Conrad-Da'Oud, 1994), suggesting a very personal engagement in learning and occurring in intimate circles of women. Viewed from the ancient tradition of women shamans, the mentor, seen as "technicians of the sacred," enable women to commune with the "more than" and heal their wounded spirits (Achterberg, 1990). Consider another story from the full moon meditation group.

A woman asked for help to claim her sense of being a woman. Estranged from her mother by death, she had never had a rite of passage to puberty. Suffering from severe endometriosis, a metaphor for her loss, she implored the women to perform a coming of age ritual. Sitting in their circle, she invoked her sense of sacred moment. Then, one-by-one, each woman whispered softly, "Here is your beauty . . . grace . . . power . . . softness," welcoming her into the fullness of her womanhood.

Third, women's groups are the setting for the celebration of the sheer "delight" in being. When women laugh, dance and sing, their spirits soar, the soul is retrieved (Arrien, 1993). Thus relieved from the oppression and silencing "out there," they are free to enjoy their womanliness, express their essential lustiness and assert their power without disapproving "eyes" to judge and condemn them (Kaschak, 1992). (See Figure 5.) These contemporary manifestations of ancient women's social world are clearly described by Judith Durek (1989):

Women knew the mysteries of life and how to invoke the primal elements of nature, touchable and untouchable. Woman passed down to woman knowledge of the elemental energies in the earth and in herself, and of how to align herself with the eternal flow of those energies, within and without.

Woman passed down to woman a sense of the primal feminine and her belonging within it. Woman passed down to woman a sense of herself as *"woman unto herself."*

Woman passed down to woman a respect for her own being, revering the Great Mother in herself and herself in the Great Mother.

Woman passed down to woman a way of being within herself as she carried out her daily tasks in which she related to herself and to the task as sacred and necessary to the completion of the cosmic cycle, to be fulfilled by her, by her alone, again and again. Through that fulfilling, she renewed the earth, blessing the cycles of nature, quietly carving into the stillness of time the steps of her repeated trips for water, her winnowing of grain, her nurturing of the earth. (p. 6)

Throughout written history the voice that ached to tell our stories has been suppressed. Today, in the vessel of their sisterhood, women are telling their prayer tales and gaining spiritual release, wholeness and courage to reclaim their birthright.

FIGURE 5. Sophia, representing the integration of feminine wisdom.

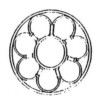

REFERENCES

Achterberg, Jeanne (1990). *Woman as healer.* Boston: Shambhala.

Achterberg, Jeanne (1993). *Working with life threatening illness.* Presentation at the Psychology of Health, Immunity and Disease Conference, Hilton Head, SC.

Allende, Isabel (1993). *Passion, authenticity, and the creative fire.* Panel discussion at the Creative Conversations Series at Quest, Grace Cathedral's Center for Spiritual Wholeness, San Francisco, CA.

Arrien, Angeles (1993). *The four fold way.* San Francisco, CA: Harper.

Arrien, Angeles (1993). *The four fold way.* San Francisco, CA: Harper.

Berne, Patricia H., & Savory, Lovis M. (1991). *Dream symbol work.* New York/ Mahwah, NJ: Paulist Press.

Bolen, Jean S. (1993a). *Ring of power.* San Francisco, CA: Harper.

Bolen, Jean S. (1993b). *Passion, authenticity, and the creative fire.* Panel discussion at the Creative Conversations Series at Quest, Grace Cathedral's Center for Spiritual Wholeness, San Francisco, CA.

Boyd-Franklin, Nancy (1991). Recurrent themes and the treatment of African-American women in group psychotherapy. *Women & Therapy, 11*(2), 25-40.

Brown, Kaaren S., & Zietfert, Marjorie (1988). Crisis resolution, competence, and empowerment: A service model for women. *Journal of Primary Prevention, 9,* (1-2) 92-103.

Chopra, Deepak (1993). *Ageless body, timeless mind.* New York: Harmony Books.

Conrad-Da'Oud, Emilie (1994). *Continuum: A brochure.* Santa Monica: Author.

Davies, Carole B. (1985). Mothering and healing in recent Black women's fiction. *Sage, 2*(1), 41-43.

Diamond, Geraldine, & Orenstein, Gloria (1990). *Reweaving the world: The emergence of ecofeminism.* San Francisco: Sierra Club.

Durek, Judith (1989). *Circle of stones: Woman's journey to herself.* San Diego: LuraMedia.

Estes, Clarissa P. (1992). *Women who run with the wolves.* New York: Ballantine Books.

Estes, Clarissa P. (1993). [Interview]. *Sounds True Catalogue Articles and Interviews, 5*(1), 29.

Frankenberg, Ruth (1993). *White women, race matters.* Minneapolis: University of Minnesota Press.

Gadon, Elinor (1992). Sacred studies for women. *New Age Journal, 9*(5), 79.

Goodman, Lisa A., Koss, Mary P., & Russo, Nancy F. (1993). Violence against women: Physical and mental health effects. Part 1: Research findings. *Applied and Preventive Psychology, 2,* 79-89.

Howa, Terry (1993). I am your witness, *New Age Journal, 10* (3), 88.

Johnson, D. W., & Johnson, F. P. (1991). *Joining together: Group theory and group skills,* 4th ed. Boston: Allyn and Bacon.

Kaschak, Ellyn (1992). *Engendered lives.* New York: Basic Books.

Kolb, David A. (1984). *Experiential learning: Experience as the source of learning and development.* Englewood Cliffs, NJ: Prentice-Hall.

Kreidler, Markelen C., & England, Diane B. (1990). Empowerment through group support: Adult women who are survivors of incest. *Journal of Family Violence, 5*(1), 35-42.

Lee, Janet (1989). "Our hearts are collectively breaking." Teaching survivors of violence. *Gender and Society, 3-4,* 541-548.

Lerner, Gerda (1986). *The creation of patriarchy.* New York: Oxford University Press.

Nelson, Mardell (1991). Empowerment of incest survivors: Speaking out. *Families-in-Society, 72* (10), 618-624.

Nelson, Jill (1993). *Volunteer slavery.* Chicago: Noble Press, Inc.

Orenstein, Gloria F. (1990). *The reflowering of the goddess.* New York: Pergamon Press.

Resnick-Sannes, Helen (1991). Shame, sexuality, and vunerability. *Women & Therapy, 11* (2), 111-125.

Ress, Mary J. (1993). Cosmic theology: Ecofeminism and panentheism. Interview with Ivone Gebara. *Creation Spirituality, 9*(6), 9-11.

Simpkinson, Anne A. (1992, July-August). In her own voice. An interview with Marion Woodman. *Common Boundary,* 22-30.

Simpkinson, Charles, & Simpkinson, Anne (1992). *Sacred stories: A celebration of the power of stories to transform and heal.* San Francisco: Harper.

Skultans, Vieda (1991). Women and affliction in Marashtra: A hydraulic model of health and illness. *Culture, Medicine and Psychiatry, 15,* 321-359.

Stone, Merlin (1990). Foreword. In G. F. Orenstein (Ed.), *The reflowering of the goddess* (pp. 9-12). New York: Pergamon Press.

Walden, Neva (1992). *Sexual abuse: A thread in the tapestry of divine sexual energy.* Presented at the International Transpersonal Association, Prague.

Walker, Alice (1993). *Passion, authenticity, and the creative fire.* Panel discussion at the Creative Conversations Series at Quest, Grace Cathedral's Center for Spiritual Wholeness, San Francisco, CA.

Woodman, Marion (1992). *Leaving my father's house.* Boston: Shambhala.

Woodman, Marion (1993). *Leaving old thresholds behind.* Presentation at the Embodying Spirit Conference, Eypsychia, Orlando, FL.

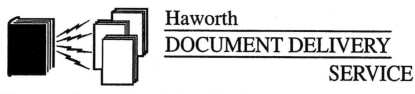

Haworth
DOCUMENT DELIVERY
SERVICE

This new service provides a single-article order form for any article from a Haworth journal.

- *Time Saving:* No running around from library to library to find a specific article.
- *Cost Effective:* All costs are kept down to a minimum.
- *Fast Delivery:* Choose from several options, including same-day FAX.
- *No Copyright Hassles:* You will be supplied by the original publisher.
- *Easy Payment:* Choose from several easy payment methods.

Open Accounts Welcome for . . .
- Library Interlibrary Loan Departments
- Library Network/Consortia Wishing to Provide Single-Article Services
- Indexing/Abstracting Services with Single Article Provision Services
- Document Provision Brokers and Freelance Information Service Providers

MAIL or *FAX* THIS ENTIRE ORDER FORM TO:

Haworth Document Delivery Service
The Haworth Press, Inc.
10 Alice Street
Binghamton, NY 13904-1580

or **FAX**: (607) 722-6362
or **CALL**: 1-800-3-HAWORTH
(1-800-342-9678; 9am-5pm EST)

PLEASE SEND ME PHOTOCOPIES OF THE FOLLOWING SINGLE ARTICLES:

1) Journal Title: _____

    Vol/Issue/Year:_____Starting & Ending Pages:_____

    Article Title:_____

_____

2) Journal Title: _____

    Vol/Issue/Year:_____Starting & Ending Pages:_____

    Article Title:_____

_____

3) Journal Title: _____

    Vol/Issue/Year:_____Starting & Ending Pages:_____

    Article Title:_____

_____

4) Journal Title: _____

    Vol/Issue/Year:_____Starting & Ending Pages:_____

    Article Title:_____

_____

(See other side for Costs and Payment Information)

COSTS: Please figure your cost to order quality copies of an article.

1. Set-up charge per article: $8.00
   ($8.00 × number of separate articles)   _____

2. Photocopying charge for each article:
   1-10 pages: $1.00   _____

   11-19 pages: $3.00   _____

   20-29 pages: $5.00   _____

   30+ pages: $2.00/10 pages   _____

3. Flexicover (optional): $2.00/article   _____

4. Postage & Handling: US: $1.00 for the first article/
   $.50 each additional article   _____

   Federal Express: $25.00   _____

   Outside US: $2.00 for first article/
   $.50 each additional article_____

5. Same-day FAX service: $.35 per page   _____

   GRAND TOTAL: _____

METHOD OF PAYMENT: (please check one)

❑ Check enclosed   ❑ Please ship and bill. PO # _____
   (sorry we can ship and bill to bookstores only! All others must pre-pay)

❑ Charge to my credit card: ❑ Visa; ❑ MasterCard; ❑ American Express;

Account Number:_____ Expiration date:_____

Signature: ✗_____

Name: _____ Institution: _____

Address: _____

_____

City: _____ State:_____ Zip:_____

Phone Number: _____ FAX Number: _____

MAIL or *FAX* THIS ENTIRE ORDER FORM TO:

Haworth Document Delivery Service	**or FAX:** (607) 722-6362
The Haworth Press, Inc.	**or CALL:** 1-800-3-HAWORTH
10 Alice Street	(1-800-342-9678; 9am-5pm EST)
Binghamton, NY 13904-1580	